Ice
Cream
in
the
Cupboard

Ice
Cream
in
the
Cupboard

PAT MOFFETT

Garrison-Savanna Publishing, LLC

Ice Cream in the Cupboard
Copyright © 2008 Pat Moffett
Published by Garrison-Savanna Publishing, LLC

For further information, please contact:
Garrison-Savanna Publishing, LLC
15 Cutter Mill Road, Suite 164
Great Neck, NY 11021

icecupboard@gmail.com

Book design by:
Arbor Books
www.arborbooks.com

Printed in Canada

Ice Cream in the Cupboard
Patrick Moffett
1. Title 2. Author 3. Memoir

Library of Congress Control Number: 2003107303
ISBN 10: 0-9742278-1-1
ISBN 13: 97809742278-1-8

This book can only be dedicated

to one person:

For Carmen

Special Thanks to:

Dr. Gisele Wolf-Klein for giving Carmen the best care possible and for her guidance and direction during this entire process.

Barbara Vogel and everyone at the Long Island Alzheimer's Foundation.

Parker Institute at Long Island Jewish Medical Center, especially **Martha Wolf** and her staff at the Granat Center.

June Herr for taking my scribbled words from that yellow paper and returning them to their rightful place in the English language.

Mia Wood for making such a difficult journey a rewarding experience. I will be forever grateful.

AUTHOR'S NOTE

When I decided to write this book I knew I wasn't going to be telling anybody anything about Alzheimer's disease that they didn't already know. Suffice it to say an Alzheimer's patient loses everything: memory, personality, ability to read, write, and even speak. This awful disease drags patients and their families through the most trying times they will ever experience.

In addition, I have not discussed the medical side of the disease. I've asked eminent geriatric specialist, Dr. Gisele Wolf-Klein, to tell you about what the future of the disease holds for Americans and patients worldwide. She writes about this and related issues in the Appendix at the end of the book.

My real mission in writing this book was to bring a renewed awareness to the category of this disease called Early Onset Alzheimer's. It's an important issue that people will have to come to grips with and, given the figures Dr. Wolf-Klein cites in the Appendix, the sooner the better. The way I've approached my mission is by telling you the story about my wife, Carmen.

She was a wonderful wife and mother who contracted Alzheimer's in her early fifties, and I knew her story would crystallize the issue of Early Onset Alzheimer's.

But before I was ready to tell this story I had to ask myself two questions. First, would Carmen approve of me writing this book? I thought about this for a while and decided that, because she always offered to help anyone less fortunate than herself, Carmen would give her blessing to the project. Second, could I be strong enough to bring back all those bad memories that I have worked so hard to rid from my mind? I knew I'd have to bring them back and relive them all over for the sake of the book, and this would be so hard to do. But when I thought about Carmen's courage in fighting this disease and her struggle to last as long as she could, I realized that writing it paled in comparison to my chore of reaching into unsafe ground.

So I suggest you sit back in your favorite reading chair. Make sure you have roll of paper towels handy, as I don't think tissues are going to be enough, and prepare to be moved like never before.

—PAT

1

That Sunday morning in June of 1998 began perfectly. Still in my pajamas, with the house to myself, I settled onto the couch to watch my favorite show, *CBS Sunday Morning* with Charles Osgood. I smiled, thinking, *What a great day. I'm not going to do anything but relax.*

My wife, Carmen, had left already to do the food shopping, which she did every Sunday morning, happily leaving me behind. Shopping wasn't my thing. I wanted to be in and out, and I always had a prepared list to speed up the process. I was the one who rushed through the store like a game show contestant who gets to keep whatever he can throw into his cart in under three minutes. Between my prepared list and my breakneck speed, having me along on a shopping trip was exhausting.

Years before, when our five kids were still living at home, I would type up the list of usual items according to their aisle number at the local supermarket in Great Neck, Long Island, where we'd lived for over twenty years. I'd add blank lines for items not on our usual list, like some steaks. Then I'd photocopy the list and hand it out at the store, giving each kid a different aisle and their own cart while Carmen and I stayed in one central location with the master cart awaiting the return of the troops. When our third little shopper dropped off their assignment, we'd get into the check out line so by the time the other two kids showed up we were ready to put their stuff on the conveyor. I remember one particular morning when we spent $280 and got the shopping done in twelve minutes flat. The kids and I were high-fiving each other over our extraordinary achievement. Carmen thought we were all nuts.

The next week, our supermarket moved the "no frills" goods from aisle two to aisle five, effectively upending my perfectly organized plan. Not only did the change destroy any chance of a pristine execution, it demolished any chance of besting last week's accomplishment.

"Excuse me, sir!" I shouted to the manager as I saw him walk by the registers. I motioned him over to where Carmen and I were waiting for our deliveries. We were a pair, Carmen and I, that's for sure. She was a slender, petite, gorgeous Puerto Rican woman, and I was a tall, formidable-looking Irish guy.

"Please tell me you're not going to ask him about the aisle change and your shopping list," Carmen implored me as the manager approached, a half smile forming on her lips. She was already edging away from my side.

"Sure," I responded. "Why not?"

"That's it! I'm disowning you. Meet me on the other side of the store." As Carmen turned to walk away, she smiled and said, "You're nutso."

Moments later, the manager was standing in front of me. "Yes sir, what can I help you with?"

"You can help me by telling me why you moved the No Frills aisle from number seven to number two," I demanded.

He cocked his head and briefly narrowed his eyes, apparently trying to figure out how I could be so upset about the change. "Well," he answered cautiously, "we thought our patrons would want to see these goods as soon as they walked in, so we moved it closer to the front entrance."

I nodded, maybe a little too rapidly, and then held up my list in front of him. "Yeah, well do you see this note?" I didn't wait for him to answer. "It's all arranged by aisle to make for faster shopping. So when you move an aisle it messes up my plan sheet." I stared at him, waiting for him to realize his error.

"I see," he said, slowly drawing out the "e." "We'll try not to do it in the future, sir."

"Great! That will be appreciated. It takes me *hours* to do this list."

As I walked away, the look on the manager's face got me thinking that maybe Carmen was right, maybe I am a little whacky.

Chuckling to myself about that memory, I stretched out on the couch for a little nap—well, I didn't stretch entirely, since the length of the couch was shorter than my six foot, two inch frame, but I still managed to doze off. The chiming of the grandfather clock awakened me soon after, however, at eleven. There was still time before Carmen would be back.

Standing to work the kinks out of my ankles from lying down, I noticed a yellow envelope propped against the family photos that sat on the fireplace mantle. The writing on the front read, "Honey." This was a good sign, because if it had said "Patrick," I would have been in deep trouble for something.

Opening the envelope, I figured it was about the night before, when Carmen and I went to our favorite restaurant in Great Neck, Gino's, where we had a nice meal at our usual corner table. It was then that we broached the subject of retirement for the first time. Carmen was a vibrant, sexy, intelligent fifty-three, and I was a still-strapping forty-eight. I always liked to razz her about robbing the cradle, and her response was always the same. "Hey, you got yourself a hot Latin woman, and I haven't seen you complaining lately." That would end the razzing. She was the most beautiful woman in the world to me. It was true.

"How about Guadalajara?" Carmen asked.

"Guadalajara?" I repeated, surprised. "Americans really retire there?"

"Yes, they do," she answered matter-of-factly. "I saw it on '60 Minutes.'"

I considered it for a moment. "I think you just want to go there because you speak Spanish and I don't."

"That's really silly."

"No, it's not. You could be making nice-nice with the mailman, and I wouldn't have a clue."

"You don't have a clue, anyway."

Carmen was always good with the comebacks. We laughed the rest of the night, polishing off our second bottle of Robert Mondavi Opus One.

Scanning the first words of the letter, I was right; the note was about the previous evening.

Honey,

I really had a wonderful time last night. "A bottle of wine, a loaf of bread and thou." Just like it's always been. I'm glad I robbed the cradle.

It was fun planning our retirement. I didn't realize we had so much to do. We raised our children well, but they're all on their own now, so the time has come for us to look to our future. I can't express all the love I have in my heart for you. You're the only man in the world for me and I'm looking forward to spending the rest of my life with you. Just remember, "Grow old with me, the best is yet to be."

Love, Me

After re-reading the letter a few times, I shook my head in awe and disbelief. Carmen's note was so moving. I couldn't believe I almost hadn't made it to our first date.

After returning from Vietnam in 1969, I went back to my job as a clerk at a Japanese ocean carrier near Wall Street. I was anxious to move into cargo sales, since that's where the real money was, but in general, I loved the import-export business.

During the next few years, I bounced around a few carriers until I landed a great job at another carrier, "K" Line. I moved up the ladder quickly, thanks to some resignations a few rungs ahead of me and some lucky breaks. It wasn't long before I was known as "Uptown Guy," because I handled the Uptown accounts on the import side like J. C. Penney, Macy's, and Sears. On the export side, Exxon, General Motors, and U. S. Steel, were among my accounts. Because I controlled so much cargo in my capacity as Uptown Guy, I never handled anything but these major accounts. "K" Line didn't want Uptown Guy distracted by smaller accounts in other territories.

That changed one sweltering summer morning. I arrived at my office at 32 Broadway a few minutes before nine. My boss, John O'Neill, was reading the overseas telexes when I walked in. As Sales Manager, he directed the activities in all the territories.

"Good morning, John," I said brightly.

He looked up and smiled. "Hey, Pat, good morning. Listen, I need you to do me a little favor."

"Sure," I replied, feeling magnanimous. "What do you need?"

"Tony B. is out sick today, and I have to follow up on a Tokyo telex. A sales lead on a company called Dodwell, Inc. 120 Wall Street."

I waited for more, hoping this wasn't really sounding like Uptown Guy was about to be sent on a mission out of his territory. Maybe all I'd have to do was make an introductory call.

"It seems Dodwell is the trading company handling a special promotion for Exxon to deliver Christmas tree lights from Hong Kong to all of their gas stations in the Caribbean that still use the Esso brand."

This didn't sound like it was going to be just a call. This didn't sound like fun at all. Then I remembered it was April 1. *This has got to be some sort of prank*, I thought.

"What?" I asked in mock disbelief. "We have an *Asia-Caribbean* service?" I couldn't help but tease him, thinking I could get in on the joke myself.

John ignored my sarcasm, and continued to fill me in on the details.

"Supposedly, the volume is estimated to be five hundred, twenty-foot containers going to Jamaica, Aruba, Barbados—

you name it. Tokyo thinks this would be perfect for our Asia-Caribbean service, but since it's controlled in New York, we've got to follow-up on the lead."

I was famous for handling automobiles, steel, chemicals, and some of the big fashion houses. But Christmas lights for gas stations? "Come on, Chief. You're killing my image here. I hope none of the other carrier reps pick up on this."

He smiled. "Listen, Mr. Cool, just go down there and see what you can find out. I have to answer to Tokyo tonight."

I knew then there was no way out. Uptown Guy was going to do some downtown business on a hot summer morning that had all the makings of becoming a hundred-degree day. "No problem," I said, trying to sound cheery about it. "I just have a few things to take care of here, but I'll head out around ten."

"Thanks, Uptown Guy. Here's the info. Dodwell's manager is a guy named Robin Stone."

I went to my desk and called over to Dodwell a few times, but got disconnected right after the operator answered each time. *Something's up with the lines*, I thought, unhappy with the prospect of a field trip. There was no way around one now.

When I left the office at ten, it was already eighty-nine degrees. Since Dodwell was only six blocks away, I decided to walk. Bad idea. It was so humid that walking felt like swimming, and I wasn't wearing trunks. Instead, I was head to ankle polyester: shirt, tie, jacket, pants, and even the socks were polyester. The only things that weren't polyester were my shoes. *Why did I give up comfort to become a fashion plate?* Little did I know, leisure suits were on the horizon.

I wallowed in the cool blast of air that hit me as I entered the lobby at 120 Wall Street. Every piece of clothing I was wearing was stuck to my skin. It took a few minutes for me to dry off, and then I checked the building directory. "21st floor, room 2100," I mumbled to myself.

I made my way to the elevator bank and got into the first open car. Right away, I noticed the walls of the car were covered on all sides with hanging pads. *Somebody's movin',* I noted as I pressed the button for the 21st floor. It went non-stop.

When the doors opened and I stepped out of the elevator, I could tell Dodwell was the company that was moving. I walked right into a traffic jam of desks and file cabinets on dollies being shoved around by moving men.

"Hey Buddy, why don't you step over where those cartons are and try to stay out of the way," he said gruffly.

"Sorry," I said and tried to nimbly make my way to that nebulous location. Behind all those cartons' I could just make out what looked like a switchboard operator behind a glass divider, busy at her PBX control panel.

"Hello?" I called out.

The window slid open and the woman took off her headset. "Can I help you?" She asked, looking slightly annoyed.

"Yes you can. Here's my card. I'm from "K" Line and I'd like to see Mr. Robin Stone."

"That's *Ronald* Stone," she corrected, and then paused before continuing. "And, no. He left the company two weeks ago."

"Okay, can you find the Traffic Manager or someone that handles transportation?" I asked.

I knew this sales call was going to be a bummer right from the beginning, I thought, frustrated.

"I'll call back there but I don't know who handles the traffic now. I'll do my best but my board has been acting up all day." She pursed her lips, frustrated at the situation.

"Yeah, I know," I said sympathetically. "I couldn't get through this morning."

Her face softened, and she gave me a hint of a smile. "It may take a few minutes. Why don't you pull up a box and sit down?"

And risk getting dust on my polyester pants? Not on your life! "That's okay, thanks." I paced around for fifteen minutes with my briefcase under my arm waiting for someone to come out.

The door finally opened and the most strikingly beautiful woman I had ever seen walked in with a purposeful stride. I swear she had a halo around her. She was petite—I guessed about 5'2"—and, from what I could tell despite her loose-fitting clothes, slender. I could see immediately that she had lips that were made for kissing, almond-shaped eyes that could melt you with a single glance, and smooth and flawless olive skin that covered high cheekbones and the classic features of a film star. *Wow. Wow. Wow.*

As she walked toward me, she fluffed her sandy blond, shoulder-length hair to get the dust out, and particles were falling on a very old Notre Dame T-shirt with a frayed neckline. The dusty shirt ended at a pair of oversized jeans with cuffs on the bottom. Topping off the ensemble was a pair of Minnetonka moccasins. They were white with those little colored beads on top. The woman was gorgeous—the outfit, tragic. But it was moving day, after all, and besides, this was a woman who could wear a paper bag and still look stunning.

I nearly lost my senses when she stopped in front of me

and looked up with an intensely direct gaze. She wasn't put off by the tall drink of water in front of her, but I was bowled over by her face. She had these deep brown eyes full of warmth. They weren't just beautiful eyes, they were eyes that reached out to you, eyes that radiated intelligence. "Hi," she said in a deep, slow voice, extending her hand. "My name is Carmen Claudio." It was the sexiest voice I'd ever heard.

Just like in the movies, time stood still for a moment as we stood holding hands. It took me a second longer to realize I should let go, but Carmen's skin was smooth, and her grip firm and assured. This, I knew, was a formidable woman.

"Well, uh," I stammered, letting go of her hand. There I was in the midst of a mess of boxes and furniture and gruff moving men, standing before a gorgeous, albeit dusty woman. *What am I doing there? Oh, yes. Business.* "I was trying to get some information on contract that Dodwell has with Exxon for Christmas tree lights going to the Caribbean." As I began talking shop, my confidence and focus returned.

"Yes," Carmen replied firmly but without a hint of hurry in her voice. "I'm familiar with that contract."

I was relieved. Maybe she could point me in the right direction. "Good, but in my position, I only speak to the Traffic Manager, not secretaries such as yourself."

Silence. The air had suddenly changed around us. Carmen narrowed her gorgeous eyes and quickly gave me the once-over. Then she breathed in deeply, as if trying to pull patience into her lungs, and brushed some more dust from her hair. Finally, she looked me straight in the eye once again. "I guess this is your lucky day, Mr. Moffett," she said with a slight Southern accent. "Because *I* am the Traffic Manager."

Silence again. I closed my eyes and shook my head. I'd just blown it in more ways than one. "Listen," I tried. "I'm really sorry, I—"

"You're damn right you're sorry," Carmen responded, eyes still narrowed, planting her hands firmly on her hips. "You're a sorry *ass!*"

She may have been petite, but she was feisty. Suddenly, I didn't feel like Uptown Guy. I was Lowdown Heel. "Carmen, I didn't mean anything by that. I was just—"

"Nonsense!" she interrupted with a graceful wave of her hand. "That's the problem today with men in our industry. They don't think a woman can handle management positions, and clearly, your attitude is indicative of that."

I shook my head, waving my hands around defensively. I backpedaled as fast as my lips could move. "No, really, we were led to believe that this position was held by a Robin Stone, a guy." I may have been a man of my generation, and may have expected a man as Traffic Manager, but I was innocent here. The name—everything—just seemed to fit.

Carmen rolled her eyes. "Lemme get my violin out for this one."

"Okay, point well taken," I said, simultaneously seeking a ceasefire and trying desperately to work my way out of the hole I'd dug for myself. "But how about this. It's a hot day today, right? I'm out of my territory, and Dodwell is moving—"

"Just to the tenth floor," Carmen interrupted.

"Fine. Only the tenth floor. In any case, things are a bit crazy today." I pulled out my business card and handed it to her. "Why don't I call you tomorrow and see if you have time for lunch. Then I can make amends for my chauvinistic behavior and we can discuss business." I held up two fingers. "Two birds, one stone."

Carmen eyed the card, pinching its edge between thumb and forefinger. It was only a few seconds, but it seemed like an hour. Finally, she looked up. I was mesmerized once again by her deep brown eyes. *Could I be falling for this woman? Is it true? Is it really love at first sight?* I never believed in that nonsense, and dismissed the thought right away. But I knew for certain I was taken by this woman.

A flutter of a smile crossed her lips, revealing perfect straight, white teeth. She said, "Tell you what. Call me tomorrow at eleven, and I'll see if I have time."

Suddenly, I was grinning ear to ear. There was no stopping it. I was a man saved from execution—and more. "Thanks, Carmen, really. I'll talk to you tomorrow." I paused a moment, then continued. "And once again, I am really sorry for the mix-up. Really."

"Yeah, yeah, yeah," she grinned. "Now get outta here so you don't mess up the moving people the way you messed up this sales call." With a wave of her hand, she disappeared behind a stack of boxes.

Smiling, I left the building and continued on with my otherwise ordinary day. Now, however, it was filled with the image and sound of this woman. Her sultry yet direct voice, her chocolate eyes, succulent lips, and silken skin…That night, I couldn't sleep for the thoughts passing through my mind over and over. I replayed Carmen so many times I had every inch, every inflection of her voice seared into my memory. I finally fell asleep with her in my mind.

In the office the next morning, I was a nervous wreck

worrying about whether or not I'd have another chance to see this woman who had, literally, become the woman of my dreams. *Would she say yes to lunch? Could I salvage the terrible impression I'd left on her? Could she possibly have any of the feelings for me as I had for her?* I tried pushing these thoughts aside and focusing on work, but every couple of minutes, my eyes were back on the clock and my mind on Carmen. It was useless.

Finally, the clock read 11:00. I grabbed the receiver and Dodwell's main line. Busy. *What?* I'd been so worried about the possibility of getting rejected by Carmen that I forgot all about yesterday's switchboard problems. I hurriedly dialed again, but no luck. Finally, on the third try, I got Dodwell's operator.

"Carmen Claudio," I said, enjoying the sound of her name.

"One moment, please. Hold on, I'll connect you."

Yes!

The phone rang twice before she answered. "Hello, this is Carmen."

Butterflies erupted in my stomach at the sound of her sultry voice. I tried sounding smooth, nonchalant. "Hi, it's Pat from K-Line. How about that lunch?"

She didn't miss a beat. "Sounds good to me, I'm starved!"

"Fine," I breathed a sigh of relief. "What time is good for you?" Already, things were looking better.

"Make it twelve-thirty," she said. "But don't come upstairs. It's still too dusty up here. Meet me in the lobby."

"OK," I said smiling. "See you there." After all the commotion, it was as simple as that. *This*, I thought, *is my kind of woman.*

120 Wall Street, like most of the financial district, was busier than it was on other days. Friday, pay day, the best day

of the week. If you were a lower-echelon employee, this was your day to shine. Dollars burning a hole in your pocket. Of course, come Monday, we were all poor slobs again, bitching about how little money we made and how our bosses sucked. But I enjoyed walking the six blocks to Carmen's building that day, and soaked up the sense of optimism that others were feeling, however fleeting.

As I made my way into her building, I had to battle the throngs on their way out for lunch. In the bustle, I found a couch just off to the left of the elevator bank, and sat down in the deep, soft cushions to wait, setting my attaché beside me. It was a relief to get 200 lbs. off my feet, and if it weren't for my excitement, I could have sat there all afternoon, relaxing and people watching. From my spot on the couch, I had a great vantage point. It was fun watching the people bolting off in various directions in search of sustenance.

Just then, the most extraordinary pair of legs making their way across the lobby caught my eyes. A pair of dark stockings covered them, and the high heels and miniskirt book-ended them to their best effect. Bodies blocked my view of the body that owned the legs, and by the time my view was unobstructed, an arch voice said, "Are you going to stare at my legs all day, or are we going to lunch?" It was Carmen. If only I'd known yesterday that those grubby jeans were covering a pair of legs as perfect as her face. *Wow*, I thought again. To say she cleaned up well would be a gross understatement. This was a woman not only with classic beauty, but also impeccable style. From head to toe, she was immaculate. Even her make-up was perfectly applied—not at all heavy—and accentuated her already lovely features.

Bumbling to extricate myself from the deep cushions, my shoes kept slipping on the shiny floor. I couldn't get any traction, and must have looked like Scooby Doo running in place, paws spinning helplessly. I made it halfway up when Carmen reached out and pulled me the rest of the way.

Reaching down for my attaché case, I mumbled, "Sorry, Carmen."

"That's two 'I'm sorrys' in as many days. Not really off to a good start, are you?" she asked matter-of-factly, but something in her eyes suggested she was enjoying the moment.

I shook my head. I just dug myself in deeper and deeper with every word. But I wasn't a quitter. I kept pitching until I got a hit. "C'mon, let's have lunch. I'll make it up to you."

I took Carmen to Delmonico's, a pricey old restaurant on Beaver Street famous with stockbrokers. They even had a stock ticker next to the bar so guys could check investments while getting hammered on their cocktail of choice.

"Vietnam," she said. "Wow."

I nodded. "You could say that. It had its moments, but let's just say I was *very* glad to come home."

"I'll bet. Everything you see on the news…" Her voice trailed off, and she looked away thoughtfully. Then she turned back to me, her face brightening. "Tell me about your family."

"Well, born and raised right here. Brooklyn."

"I gathered as much," she laughed.

"Whaddya mean?" I said in mock horror, laying on the thickest accent I could muster.

She just laughed and raised her eyebrows.

"I guess that says it all," I laughed with her. "Well, let's see.

No brothers or sisters. Family still here, thankfully, grandparents, too. Your turn."

"Oh, let's see," she said, smoothing her skirt. "Born in Caguas, Puerto Rico. Beautiful place. My family moved to Fayetteville, North Carolina, where Fort Bragg is, when I was a one-year old, and I grew up there."

"Huh. I thought I heard a little Southern hint in there."

She shrugged. "Yeah, I missed the accent mostly—but I can find it at a moment's notice. What else? My parents died when I was a teenager."

"Oh," I said, sad to hear that they were lost to her so young. It explained her strength. "I'm sorry."

"I had my sisters, though, Millie and Evelyn. And my brother, J.R. There was family all around. We were a pretty tight-knit group. My uncles and cousins were in the 82nd Airborne Division at Fort Bragg. They're all paratroopers."

Well, I thought, *If it works out with Carmen, the family get-togethers should be interesting, since I'm a leg.* During my time in the military I was with the rival 101st Airborne Division.

Carmen continued telling me about her family. "And now I've got three beautiful girls, too, Lisa, Lesly, and Laura." She must have seen the look on my face because she quickly added, "Divorced."

"Me, too. But no kids."

After two hours of talking over a great lunch, it was time to head back to work. As we left the restaurant, I realized we'd talked about everything under the sun—except the all-important Exxon Christmas tree lights headed for the Caribbean.

"Say, Carmen, we've got ships calling at all the ports you need for the Exxon distribution, and the best rates available."

"I know," she replied. "You got the business."

Quick decision, I thought, but I wasn't going to complain.

After that, there were many lunches, which led to numerous cocktails, followed by quite a few dinners, which, in turn, led to weekend getaways. Before we knew it, we were joined at the hip. My only concern as we were falling in love was that I didn't know what my fatherly role would be. Carmen's three daughters were young, and the eldest, Lisa, was very close with her father. How would I fit in? "I don't know how to be a father, let alone one to three young girls," I told Carmen.

"Listen," she said, reaching up to touch my face. She smiled, and her eyes reached out to me with more love than I had ever felt in my life. "My children will love you the way I love you."

I never asked a thing after that. Ever. And then Carmen Claudio, the most beautiful woman in the world married me, and life was sweet.

We were a perfect pair, best friends with a great romance. "We're the last of the great romantics," Carmen would whisper in my ear as we danced in our small living room, at the Great Neck Terrace apartments. We both loved to dance, and would make a date on a weekend night, just the two of us. The girls would be at a sleepover, and we would have a night to ourselves. We'd order in, have a bottle of wine, and play everything from The Stylistics to Sinatra. It was a grand time, and I had an amazing dance partner.

Even our conflicts, both minor and major, reflected a partnership achievable, so far as I'm concerned, only by people who genuinely like and respect each other. I grew as a man because I had a partner who could challenge and support me. For example, one day during our courtship, a woman stopped me in Manhattan who was seeking directions to the Union Square subway station.

Well, I thought. *I can handle this. After all, I've got a Spanish-speaking girlfriend.* I leaned down, and in my best Spanish accent, I bellowed, "El blocko ocho avenita subterraneo Union Square."

As I spoke, the woman slowly recoiled, her eyes widening in confusion. She opened her mouth, then apparently decided otherwise, and just smiled. "Okay."

Later, I told Carmen about my civic and linguistic achievement. "You *what?*" she exclaimed, planting her hands firmly on her hips. "Oh, man. You fractured it—no, you *broke* the language."

"Whaddya talking about?" I spread my arms wide, palms up. "I helped the woman out."

"Really. I'll bet she's still wandering around Manhattan looking for the station. You don't learn Spanish by osmosis, you know." Then she turned her head slightly, examining my face. "Do you know how good you've got it with me?" she asked rhetorically.

She was right, and I knew it. I always knew it. I would have my share of successes over the years, it was true, but none of it would have been possible without Carmen. I wouldn't have made it without her. When, years later, I made vice president, I half-jokingly yelled, "I'm vice president of the world!" I was proud of myself and, as a driven and self-made man, found great self-worth in career advancement.

But Carmen wouldn't let it go to my head too much. "Okay, Mr. International, take out the garbage." The sweetest woman in the world was also *nobody's* pushover—but she was also the most supportive.

"You should write a book," she declared one night. We'd been talking about my experiences in Vietnam. I wasn't one to talk much about it, but somehow, we'd found ourselves on the topic. I regaled her with stories of a military mix-up that probably saved my life, rescuing orphans, and the madness of surviving it all.

"I wouldn't have wanted to know you then," she said quietly. "Not knowing where and how you were...that would have been too much."

"Then we're lucky," I said. "Because here we are, together now."

2

As my daydreaming about the early days with Carmen came to a close, I glanced at the clock. "12:45." Even for my slow-poke shopper, Carmen, this was much later than usual.

Dragging my butt off the couch, I went to the front windows and looked outside. I was half-expecting to see Carmen roll up the driveway that very moment, but our residential street was quiet. I gazed out the window for a few more minutes, but no Carmen appeared. As I started to turn away, a car caught the corner of my eye. I looked closer, and saw it was a familiar-looking gray Camry turning right from Westminster Avenue onto our street, Pembroke Avenue. *Oh, good, there she is.* But instead of turning into our driveway, the car rolled right by. *Strange. Looked like Carmen's Camry. Maybe it wasn't.* The car was speeding along, so between that and the sycamore tree and sunlight in my eyes, I hadn't got a look at the driver. I figured it was just a coincidence, and kept my lookout for Carmen.

A few minutes later, what looked like the same car turned the corner onto our street again, and sped by the house. But this time, I clearly saw it was my Carmen. *What the heck?* It wasn't long before the car turned a third time onto our street, but this time, Carmen came straight into the driveway.

I went outside to help with the bags, but before I even got a chance to open the car door, I heard her yelling at the top of her lungs, "It'd be nice if someone *got off their ass* and helped me!"

"Carmen, calm down. I'm right here." It wasn't like Carmen to be mercurial. She had a fiery temper at times, but she wasn't one of those people who went off out of the blue.

"*Calm down* my ass," she snapped. "Pick up these bundles and get them in the house."

Carrying the grocery bags inside, I tried to figure out why she was so agitated. "Hey, hon?" I called back. She was busying herself with some bags. "Not for nothing, but why did you drive by the house twice before pulling in?"

"What? That wasn't *me*." Her tone of voice was disdainful, as if I had said the most ridiculous thing in the world. I stopped to look back at her. Then she continued, rummaging through her purse in frustration. "It was probably another Camry that just *looked* like mine."

"No," I shook my head in confusion. "It was you because—"

"I *said*," she interrupted, looking at me. Her voice was icy. "It *wasn't* me. *End* of story."

I looked at her a moment before deciding not to pursue the issue. *Maybe she's got her period worse than usual,* I thought. Whatever it was, something was not right.

Everything for us had begun perfectly. When Carmen and I married and moved into the Great Neck Terrace apartments, we already had an instant family. Her three girls became mine, too. There was Lisa, who was ten, and twins Lesly and Laura, who were six. Later, we would have two boys together, P.J. and Craig.

The transition was especially hard for Lisa, and she would often decide to go live with her father for periods of time before she got homesick and changed her mind. But overall, things were smooth, and we formed a cohesive family. Laura was an academically minded child from an early age, and Lesly was a terrific athlete. Things just clicked for us, and even though we struggled financially, we made it work. We both worked full time jobs, and on top of that, I went to night school, and Carmen cared for the kids. We got through because Carmen was a master of budgeting, and she always managed to make everything simple feel like a grand event. Whether it was preparing traditional Puerto Rican dishes with exquisite flair, or darning the kids' clothes to give them new life, Carmen could make everything beautiful.

Not long into our marriage, Carmen announced she was pregnant. I was elated, and promptly tried to get Carmen to sit down and put her feet up.

"Oh, stop that nonsense," she playfully scolded me. "I'm made of peasant stock and we're stronger than that. However," she added with a wry smile, "you may lavish me with undying love and attention." Needless to say, Carmen was thrilled. She adored children, and the chance to have more was a gift.

"Deal."

I wanted to be a part of the entire process, and so we agreed to take a Lamaze class together when she got to seven months. A nurse over in nearby Port Washington was conducting some sessions at her house, and we eagerly signed up.

The first night, there were ten couples. We all sat in a large circle, the women sitting on the pillows they'd brought, and the men sitting just in front of each of their partners.

"Okay," the nurse announced. "We're going to start with some breathing exercises." She looked at me. "Mr. Moffett, I've got a special role for you."

"I'm ready," I replied.

"You're going to play the part of the contraction," she said, winding up a large children's clock that had a big second hand. Then she passed it to me. "Every time the hand hits twelve, you raise your hand and yell, "Contraction!" That will be everyone's cue to begin the breathing exercise."

Carmen burst out laughing. Leaning forward, she said, "Certainly not one of your more famous roles, is it dear?"

I had to laugh, too. "Yeah, yeah. Now, shut up and breathe."

That was the first and last fun we had with Lamaze. Carmen developed a life threatening condition called Placenta Previa, in which the placenta sits on top of the cervix, thereby blocking it.

One night after school, I came home to find a note on the door: "Don't go inside. Come to my house right away.—Bob." *Don't go into my own apartment?* I thought angrily. *I don't think so.* I walked in the door. The apartment was dark and empty. Then I saw the blood, a tremendous amount of blood. Carmen's clothes, which were scattered on the floor, were soaked—shoes, pants, under clothes.

I ran next door to our neighbors, Nellie and Bob Gladd. "What's happened?" I asked, though somehow I already knew it had to do with the pregnancy.

"Carmen called over earlier and Nellie drove her to the hospital. Carmen was hemorrhaging—it was—"

He didn't get a chance to complete the sentence, because I turned and starting racing over to my car. "Let's go!" I yelled. We sped to the hospital, where we waited for news. Carmen was being prepped for an emergency Caesarean section, but I had to wait to see her.

Bob paced anxiously in the waiting room in the maternity ward. "Bob," I said in exasperation. "Why don't you sit the fuck down already?"

"I can't," he replied, his expression pained. "I'm too nervous."

He was. So nervous, in fact, that a nurse came over to him and said, "Don't worry, Sir, she'll be okay."

"I'm not the father, it's him!" he exclaimed, pointing to me.

Bob didn't have kids, so he had no idea what pregnancy was all about. I looked at him, thinking he was going to faint any second.

Just then, the elevator doors opened and about a half dozen guys walked out carrying Lamaze bags. "They look like the Montreal Canadians," he said. Then we both laughed, relaxing for a moment.

That levity was broken when a nurse came out to tell me I could see Carmen for a moment before the surgery began.

I had only enough time to give her a kiss and tell her I loved her before I was ushered out. She was just barely going under from the anesthesia when they began the surgery.

Later I learned that Carmen had started hemorrhaging so severely that if she had got to the hospital just twenty minutes later than she did, she would have died.

A while later, I was introduced to P.J., my son. I couldn't hold him because he was in an incubator. His skin was jaundiced, and they were keeping him under warm lights until he recovered. But I stared at him endlessly, marveling at his perfection.

Carmen was completely out of it for a couple of days, and was kept at the hospital for eight days before being released. In the meantime, I went every day and held and fed P.J., and got to be with Carmen when she met her son for the first time. Thankfully, Carmen made a full recovery, and later joked about getting our money back from the Lamaze classes.

Soon after our first son, P.J. was born in 1976, it became apparent that we'd outgrown our two-bedroom apartment in Great Neck. It was time to take the plunge and go into debt like the rest of America. It was time, in other words, to buy a house.

Carmen and I spent weekend after weekend scouring Long Island looking for the right house for our brood. My mom had passed away during the winter and left me a few dollars from her company's insurance policy. Carmen and I decided to apply most of this money as a down payment on a new home. That was the simple part. Finding a suitable place to live and raise our children wasn't.

Three weeks and about twenty houses later, we were starting to become disillusioned and frustrated. Nothing caught our attention. We decided to take a "life" break and forego house hunting for a while. It had been a few years since we'd had a vacation, and thought a trip to Disney World would be the perfect family holiday. It would be particularly special for the girls, who never complained about not having all the toys all the other kids had. We just could never afford them before. But this trip would make up for that.

First, however, we had to get a new car. My 1968 Pontiac Bonneville had 90,000 miles on it, and was gasping toward its last breath. Carmen's car was a clunker, too. So, on a bright and warm May Saturday morning, the family sat at the table and planned out the day's chores over breakfast. Carmen would head off to the beauty parlor for the works—haircut and color, manicure, and pedicure. The girls would do some household chores, and P.J. would accompany me to the travel agent on Northern Boulevard and the Chevy dealership in Douglaston, Queens.

By the time we set out, it was already seventy degrees and perfect for car buying. First, we went to the travel agent, where I picked out a good family package to the Magic Kingdom, scheduling the trip for later that summer. Then P.J. and I made our way over to the Bay Chevrolet dealer.

As soon as we entered the showroom, I saw it: a bronze Chevy Malibu with a dark brown vinyl top. It sat in the center of the showroom floor, and I was immediately drawn to it. The inside had an inviting tan leather interior, and it wasn't ten seconds before I slid behind the wheel, cradling P.J. on my lap. I was surrounded by that "new car" smell that makes it so difficult to walk away. As I scanned the dash, I saw the odometer showed the car already had 150 miles. Then I noticed the "Demo" sign hanging from the rearview mirror.

"Great little set of wheels, isn't she?" a voice boomed next to my ear.

Startled, I looked up to see a salesman's face about six inches from mine. "Yes, yes, it really is nice," I agreed. I moved to open the door and get out. "But it looks like it'll be out of my price range, anyway."

"Son, this is a demo, which means I got a lot of latitude to cut you a sweet deal on this baby." He waited for me to organize P.J. in my arms before extending his hand. "By the way, my name is Sal."

I shook his hand, and introduced myself. "My name's Pat, and this is my son, P.J."

Sal looked down at P.J. and smiled. "Well, isn't he cute," Sal said, patting P.J. on the head.

"He sure is," I responded proudly. One of P.J.'s many good qualities was that he didn't fuss when others wanted to touch or hold him—and he never barfed on anybody in the process.

After Sal made some *goo goo, ga ga* noises, I got back to business. "Anyway, what's a demo?"

"Well son, we need cars to take out on the road for potential customers to test drive. The salesmen get to drive these cars for their own personal use as well. I myself drove this little Malibu so I know it's a terrific car."

I nodded, and took a stroll around my potential new car, looking for any dings. It was immaculate.

"C'mon," Sal said, gesturing me over with a wave of his hand. "Let's talk some numbers."

I followed him into his cubicle and sat down. He walked behind his desk and jotted some numbers on a piece of paper. Then he slid it across the desk to me.

It was much lower than I was expecting. Trying to control my growing excitement, I crossed out his number and jotted down one of my own in response. I figured that it couldn't hurt to haggle. I slid the paper back to Sal.

"Deal!"

I was thrilled. I gave Sal a down payment in cash and filled out the paperwork for the car loan with GMAC. He told me it would be ready on Monday evening but that I should call first to make sure it was ready. What he really meant was "Don't come by if the loan doesn't go through." But I was sure it would. Feeling pretty good about myself, I grabbed P.J., shook hands with Sal, and left for home. It was a good day: I got a good price to take the family to the Magic Kingdom and negotiated a great price for an almost new car. Now it was time to sit back and relax.

Back at home, I settled P.J. into his high chair in front of the television, and got him some Beech Nut strained peas. Then I made myself a ham sandwich, got a Coke, and joined P.J. in the living room. After feeding him, I turned my attention to the first inning of the Mets game against the Cardinals at Shea Stadium. The day was getting better and better. But just as I was about to bite into my sandwich, the phone rang. *Damn.* I put everything down on the coffee table and went to the kitchen.

"Hello," I said in an unfriendly tone.

"Hello, it's me." Carmen. Immediately, I softened. Ever since Todd Rundgren came out with a song of the same name, it was Carmen's trademark phone greeting.

"Are you done already?" I asked.

"No, not quite, but I have something to tell you."

"Shoot."

"You know Danny, my hairdresser?"

"Not intimately." I looked longingly in the direction of my sandwich.

"Stop kidding. This is important."

"Sorry," I said, my attention snapping back to my wife's voice. "Go ahead."

"He just told me that he and his wife are getting a divorce!"

"He's married?! I thought he was gay."

"That's the problem with you guys from Brooklyn," she sniffed. "You think all hairdressers are gay."

"So that's what was so important?" I asked teasingly.

"No! But Danny and his wife are selling their house and the sooner it sells the sooner they can part company."

"Okay, go on."

"The house is right here in Great Neck, on Pembroke Avenue," she said, her tone becoming more excited. "I think that's the street that we pass as a short cut to the expressway."

"Yeah, I think I know the street. Anyway, what do we do now?" I knew she had dreams of moving before we had even laid eyes on the house. There was nothing to do at this point except follow along and see what happened.

"Well Danny suggested that I go to the house and knock on the door, that I should meet his wife Anna without making any reference to knowing him because the divorce is so nasty. He said I should give her the story that we don't have much money with kids to raise, and see what happens."

I paused for a moment to be sure she was finished with her story. "Carmen, frankly speaking, you're not so far away with the poor approach." I hated to be a downer, but it was true.

"I know but what do you think of the idea?"

"Fine, Carmen," I agreed. "Go ahead but just don't put a binder on the house."

Her voice was ebullient. "I agree. No problem!"

We hung up, and I went back to watching the Met game with P.J. After about an hour the phone rang again.

"Hello," I answered cautiously.

"Hello, It's Me."

"Hi, How did it go?"

"It went great!" Then there was a pause before she added, "And I put a binder on it."

I practically jumped out of my skin. "*What?* I thought we agreed to no binders!"

"I know," she said, "But as soon as I walked in the house, I knew it was perfect for us." Before I could bust a gasket, she said hurriedly," I already worked out a budget for us so we can swing the payments."

It occurred to me just then that Carmen was no longer at the house, but I didn't know where she was. "Where are you calling from anyway?" We didn't have cell phones, of course, in those days.

"A phone booth in the Shell station on Northern Blvd." She said matter-of-factly.

"So you worked out an entire budget for our foreseeable future in a phone booth?"

Ignoring me, she said, "Listen, I'm on my way home. Just be patient until I can explain."

I shook my head, but couldn't help grinning at my wife's pluck. "I can hardly wait." That was Carmen, a can-do, optimistic woman. There was never anything that Carmen couldn't get done once she set her mind to it.

About ten minutes later, Carmen came walking in the door holding a bottle of Chivas Regal scotch over her head. "Peace offering?" she asked smilingly.

"Honey, I'm not mad. I'm just concerned that we won't be able to pull off buying a house, buying a car and going to

Disney World all at one time," I protested. "Besides, I didn't go to bed as myself and wake up as J.P. Morgan."

"Let me show you," she said, and traded the scotch for a yellow legal pad sitting on the living room desk. I moved to the kitchen to put ice in two glasses. Then I poured us both a couple of Chivas on the rocks. For the rest of the day, we crunched numbers. When it was all over, I knew I had to go see the house.

I fell in love with it right away. It wasn't much to look at, but it was going to be ours forever. Two stories, with a nice backyard, I could almost hear the white, small Colonial style house calling to me: "Buy me and you won't be sorry." I was hooked, and the house was right, I wasn't sorry. We'd have to put off Disneyland for a little while, but the house would more than make up for it.

Soon enough, we were settled in at our new home on Pembroke Avenue. Lisa called it "1313 Mockingbird Lane," after the television series, *The Munsters*. It was true, the house was in dire need of repair. I guess you could call it a "handyman special." I, however, was anything but handy. If I had to put a screw into the wall, I'd stare at a hammer, pliers, and a screwdriver trying to figure out which one to use. But, I was staring at objects in my own house, and that made all the difference.

Carmen's budget worked out as usual. We ate a lot of pasta dinners, but we made it work, and were able to raise our family in that house for over twenty years. It wasn't without its ups and downs, but we always got through.

3

By the early 1980s, after having worked my way steadily for four years toward the top of the corporate ladder at Audiovox, the payoff was in sight. If I kept at it long and hard enough, I would make it to the top of the corporate ladder. I was Traffic Manager, and needless to say, the job took all my attention. The company was growing, and demanded all of my time. The workday didn't end at five, but often continued on at a nearby bar or restaurant to entertain clients. I was in by eight and barely had time for a ham sandwich over the next ten or twelve hours, the pace was so grueling. Of course, all of this meant I didn't give much to my family beyond a growing pay-check, and it took its toll.

I was tired from giving my all at the office, and wasn't really available for much at home. Carmen and I argued more and more. Often, I didn't call home to say I was coming home late—and coming home late was almost a nightly habit. Weekends were spent trying to recover, and so Carmen was left most often to spend most of that time with the kids and household errands.

On top of that, Carmen was busy working, too. She'd never really stopped. In fact, three months after P. J. was born, Carmen had gone back to work in the same position as before, but with another firm. She was a crackerjack in so many ways, a working mother who managed to do *everything* with remarkable grace and style. Somehow, she made everything she did look effortless. But the hectic pace of our individual lives put a strain on our relationship.

One night, Carmen sat me down at the dining table. "We can't be like this," she told me, taking my hand.

"Yeah, I know," I responded. "You're right."

But nothing changed. My hard-driving work life continued unabated for another couple of years. Finally, Carmen couldn't take it anymore. She stood in the front hall as I walked in the door. "I want a divorce."

Without batting an eye, I said, "Fine, if that's what you want." No matter how muddleheaded my thinking at the time was, and no matter how crazy I was to even think of letting the best woman for me go, the fact was, I was a driven Irishman from Brooklyn. It was as if I wasn't going to be bested at home anymore than I was at work. I was competitive through and through. "I don't think that solves anything here—"

The look on Carmen's face stopped me. She'd had enough. There was no point in talking anymore. "Okay," where will you go?"

"Me? I'm not going anywhere. You want out, then you're out." She didn't argue with me. After all, it was my mom's money that got us into this house, and it felt like she was there. I wasn't going to leave that. "I'll buy you out," I offered. It would be a good deal. The house was still in disrepair. With five kids, two of them rambunctious young boys, we never really had the opportunity to put everything together.

Carmen agreed, and spent the next several weekends looking for a place. It was a given the kids would go with her, but I wasn't happy about it. Although Lisa was already twenty, the twins, at sixteen, were still in high school, and the boys were so young, only eight and six. Eventually, Carmen found an apartment in Queens. Before I knew it, they were all gone.

The day before Carmen and the kids moved, friends of ours in eastern Long Island called to invite me to spend the day with them. "Come on," Jerry told me. "What are you gonna do all day? It'll just be awkward, and you'll feel in the way. Come stay with us."

I agreed, and got up early the next morning to be at Jerry and Lynn's house for breakfast. What I really wanted was a beer. Lynn met me at the door and ushered me in like a mother hen. "We'll get a good breakfast in you, and you'll feel better."

"Thanks," I muttered. "Thanks."

"Looks like rain, huh," Jerry greeted me.

I made a sorry stab at humor. "I'm bringing it with me."

He patted me on the back. "That's March for you. At least you didn't bring the snows of February back."

Things started off well. The coffee was hot and strong, and sitting in my friends' kitchen actually felt comfortable, rather than the ugly reminder of what I was losing I was expecting. That didn't last long.

"Scrambled or fried?" Jerry asked.

"Anything's fine, really," I answered.

I sat at the kitchen table as Jerry and Lynn worked around at the counter and stovetop, she squeezing oranges, and he getting the grill ready for a hearty meal.

"Anything it is," Jerry said brightly, turning to the fridge for eggs.

"Right," Lynn muttered. "Anything."

Jerry slammed the refrigerator door, and wheeled around. "What is *that* supposed to mean?"

"Nothing, nothing," Lynn chirped.

"Oh, please."

"If this is a bad time," I said, "I can come back later."

Lynn, without missing a beat, said, "Oh, you men. Always coming back later." Then she continued cracking eggs into a large bowl with great enthusiasm.

"Dammit, Lynn!" Jerry yelled. "Why don't you just come out and say it."

Lynn remained silent as she beat the eggs, so Jerry looked at me. "I came home late last night—"

"Again," Lynn interjected.

"*I'm* telling this story. You had your chance."

"So did you."

Jerry heaved a sigh and continued. "Anyway, she's peeved because I came home late smelling of a touch of alcohol. So what? I work hard. I have a drink. What's the problem?"

"The *problem*," Lynn said loudly as she poured the egg mix into a skillet. "The problem is that it's not the first time, and the smell ain't just alcohol."

Increasingly uncomfortable, I started to get up. "I don't

want you guys to go through all the trouble of breakfast just for me—"

"No! Sit down," Lynn exclaimed. Then she added softly, "Please."

"I just don't want to be in the way."

"*You're* not in the way," Lynn said, casting dagger eyes at Jerry. Then she went back to her eggs while Jerry made us up some Bloody Marys.

Breakfast was good, but there was still tension in the room. Soon enough, they started back in on each other and the pitch was enough to blast my eardrums.

Finally, I found my chance to interject. "Look, um, I appreciate the breakfast, but I'm gonna go. I'll be fine on my own. Really."

They didn't try to talk me out of it, and I headed out. By now, it was pouring rain, and I began to ache, physically feel sick to my stomach. *What happened? Where did things go wrong?* Carmen, the love of my life, was leaving me. We'd decided on a legal separation instead of initiating divorce proceedings right away, but it didn't make me feel any better.

I climbed into my car and started driving south on the Wantagh Parkway with no particular destination in mind. I switched on the radio absentmindedly, hoping to get my mind off my situation. Shirley Bassey was singing Neil Sadaka's, "The Hungry Years." It was a song both Carmen and I loved. "We made it through the top/We went so hard we couldn't stop/We never realized the price we had to pay." I had to turn it off. Then I saw the exit for Jones Beach.

The beach was empty. I pulled my Cadillac into the giant desolate parking lot, and parked facing the water. For a minute or two I thought I'd get out and walk the boardwalk, think about things. But I didn't have the energy. Instead, I rested my forehead against the steering wheel and closed my eyes, just to block it all out.

I don't know how long I was there when the cop rapped on my window. I jumped out of my seat, and quickly regained my composure. The windows were pretty fogged up, so it wasn't until I rolled down my window that I saw it was state park police officer.

"You all right sir?" he asked, leaning over in the rain.

"Yes, yes, officer, I'm fine. I just lost track of time."

He inspected me for a moment. "I hope you weren't drinking any alcohol."

"No. Just coffee earlier." I paused a moment. "It's just. Today, my wife is moving out. I had nowhere else to go, and I just wanted a little quiet."

He held up his hand. "It's okay, I understand. You take your time."

"Thanks, officer."

Then I was alone again. The rain lightened up a bit, so I walked around a while. By the time I got back to the car, it was three in the afternoon, and I figured safe to return home.

When I walked in the door, the silence was deafening. For a long while, I stood in the front hall, waiting for something to happen. Waiting for a familiar noise. Nothing. At that moment, I knew I was utterly alone.

Immediately, I missed the life that Carmen and the kids brought to the place. Each one of the children's unique personalities hung in the air. Lesly and Laura, though twins, were remarkably different in both physical appearance and temperament. Laura was tall, serious, and a consistently straight A student, while Lesly was petite and thin like her mom, bubbly, vivacious, and athletic. P.J. was already developing a love of planes, just like me, and was a great little athlete. Craig, who had serious health issues as an infant, was growing into a healthy, energetic little boy. Carmen had been a pillar of motherhood during his illness, which had taken us by surprise. Now, as I stood in the living room, the shock of their absence hit me like a ton of bricks.

I took the separation hard, blaming myself for Carmen leaving me. For a long time, it was all I could do to go to work and come home at the end of the day to the empty house. I did get to see the kids on weekends, and of course kept up with child support, but nothing was the same. After picking them up on Thursdays, we'd try to cobble together a normal weekend, but on Sunday evenings, I was alone again. The conversations Carmen and I had were cordial, but brief.

I made a few stabs at seeing more of Carmen. I invited her to see "Dreamgirls" on Broadway—we'd both been avid theatergoers together—but the show was so loud we left before the second act. As much as it pained me, it seemed more and more that we just weren't meant to get back together.

After a couple of years, I finally started seeing someone. It was Linda, an old friend of Carmen's from the industry. Actually we started dating by accident.

I had a shipment of cordless phones coming in to NY, but a guy in Miami was buying them, so I was supposed to go down and finish the deal. That's when I remembered Linda.

I called Carmen. "Is Linda still in Miami? If she is, I want to get her help on a deal—save me a trip."

"Yeah, sure. I've got her number. Hold on."

Within minutes, I was on the phone with Linda, and only about a minute after that, I also had a date.

"Linda, hi. Pat Moffett. How are you?"

"Pat? Well, hello! It's so good to hear from you. How's Carmen?"

"Oh, well, uh, we're not. We're separated."

"*Really*?" her voice rose at the end of the word, signaling interest. "That's too bad."

"Yes, yes it is. Listen, I'm actually calling on business. I—"

"If you're coming into town, let me know. We'll have drinks. I always did like you."

You had to hand it to Linda. She was direct. In the end, I decided to head down to Miami anyway, finish the deal myself, and see Linda. That's how it started.

We saw each other about once a month, often less than that. On some weekends, if I didn't have the kids, I'd go to Miami or she'd come up to New York. It was fun, easy. Linda was good company, and I was grateful for that. Eventually, however, Linda felt like she had to tell Carmen. She thought it was somehow dishonest to be dating her friend's husband, even if we were separated.

The next time Linda came to New York, she went to visit Carmen. It didn't go well. Carmen was furious. I could have sworn I heard her screaming and yelling all the way from Queens.

Carmen and I didn't talk for a long time after that. The girls weren't pleased with me, either, and our relationship cooled. I tried to explain to them just how lonely I was, and apologized for hurting them, but things were strained between us. They felt I'd betrayed their mom.

When Carmen cooled down, we started talking again, and even took the boys to Disneyworld, just as we'd planned to do before we bought our house. It was wonderful. Even though P. J. got sick with the flu and we had to return early, it felt like family again. Carmen even started talking about moving back. It was then that I realized that Carmen wasn't about to lose her husband to another woman, and certainly not to her friend.

Eventually, Lisa got pregnant, and that really brought us back together. She was living with Carmen, and it became clear that the relationship with the father was not going to result in marriage. I called Carmen to see if I could help ease some of the stress. "C'mon," I pressed. "Let me take you to dinner. Just us, some wine. It'll give you a chance to decompress."

She agreed, and we had a terrific evening at The Rafters. Looking at my beautiful wife, I knew I did not want to lose her for good. I may have been stubborn, but I wasn't stupid— at least not anymore. Everything about her was both familiar and exciting, from her precocious and razor-sharp wit and intellect to her short sandy blonde hair, those rich almond eyes and ruby red lips, and right down to her perfectly manicured toes. She was the mother of my children and my best friend. This was the woman I had always loved and admired. I could not let her go.

Carmen and I started spending more and more time together, and I talked about fixing up the bedroom for Lisa to have during her pregnancy. By this time, too, I knew that Linda and I were not going to last. At another Rafters dinner, I told Carmen we had to give it another chance. "Listen, I don't think you found anybody that you could say was better than

PAT MOFFETT

me, and I can't find anybody better than you, so I think we're really stuck with each other."

She looked at me for a long moment, her deep brown eyes smiling. "I agree. Let's go. What's the date? I'm ready."

We'd been talking around it for weeks, but never said the words. Now it was real. The family would be back together in time for Christmas.

"This time, we go back to the things that made us happy," she said. "The things that were just for us."

I agreed. Friday night dancing would be resurrected.

The boys were over the moon about it. On December 10th, 1988, they moved back in. The house was once again whole. Soon enough, we had an addition to the family. Lisa's daughter, Meghan, was born.

44

4

We knew we wanted to make changes. Carmen was determined to spend more time at home with the boys. She'd been
in import-export at Mitsubishi, but it hadn't gone well. The
commute to Manhattan was a grind, as were the hours. And,
as one of only a few women there, she felt isolated. "Dad,"
she said shortly after we got back together. She had early on
got into the habit of calling me "Dad," which I learned came
from her Puerto Rican background where even fathers call
their sons "Dad" as a term of respect and endearment.
"Listen, I found something. It's at Lakeville Elementary. A
typist position. I'll be right down the street—much closer to
home for the kids."

I was taken aback, at first. Carmen had always been a high-
powered manager, and the Lakeville position was far beneath
her managerial skills. Not only that, it would pinch our wal-
lets, as the position would pay significantly less than Carmen
had been used to making. Still, it would give her proximity to

the boys, and more time to spend with them. Carmen had always loved all children, not just her own, and this would give her the chance to be around them more often. Besides, there was an increasing number of Spanish-speaking families moving into the area, Carmen would often have the opportunity to work as a translator for parents who weren't bilingual. I instantly agreed, and we began organizing our reunited lives.

Soon after Carmen, Lisa, and the boys had settled in, I had to go down to Rio de Janeiro for five days on business. I knew I wanted to bring back something special for Carmen. Fortunately, I was traveling with my colleague, Frank. He was a quintessential New York Italian who knew several jewelers in the Rio area. Peter was with us, too, a big guy who spoke fluent Spanish and could translate when I was ready to make a deal. "Don't worry," Frank told me in his thick Brooklyn accent. "I'll get you quality. Tell me what she likes."

"Amethysts. It's her favorite stone. And it's got to be something really unique. My wife collects antique jewelry, so she knows her stuff."

He waved me off. "Don't worry. I know exactly where to go."

Frank took us to a store somewhere deep in the city. Standing around a table in a store, we started inspecting rocks. Everything looked so expensive. "Frank, this is too much. I can't afford this."

"Don't worry," he shook his head. "Just wait."

Then a man pulled out a dark velvet bag, and opened it. Large, uncut amethysts spilled out onto the table. "Frank, these are amazing, but come on."

"Pick one out," Frank commanded.

I looked over the stones until my eyes rested on one with a remarkable shape. I picked it up, and held it to the light. It looked like a heart.

Frank leaned over. "Yes, that one is lovely."

"But it's huge. I can't afford this!"

"Just a moment." He turned to Peter. "Ask the guy what sort of deal we can get."

Peter and the man started haggling in Spanish.

As I waited, I turned the naturally beautiful stone over in my hand. This would be the perfect gift for Carmen, if only...

Peter put a meaty hand on my shoulder. "This guy's saying that if you buy the setting, you can have the stone. It's one hundred fifty, U.S. The setting is nice, too."

I turned to Frank, who nodded sagely. It was a deal. When I returned to pick up the piece before I left Rio, I was impressed. The setting was a beautiful, rich gold, with a solid chain to match. It would look lovely on Carmen.

Flying home with the amethyst in my pocket, I thought, *We made it this far. Now, the best is yet to come.*

The next weekend, Carmen and I arranged to have the house to ourselves for an evening. We lit the fire, ordered in Italian, and popped a bottle of Merlot. With the lights dimmed and Sinatra's "What Are You Doing The Rest Of Your Life?" spinning on the record player, we lounged on pillows in front of the fire. *I want to see your face in every kind of light...*

I almost felt nervous as I slipped my hand into my pocket for the jewelry box, as if I was once again about to slip a ring on this lovely woman's finger. "For you," I said, smiling. *What are you doing for the rest of your life? North and South and East and West of your life?*

Carmen's face lit up. "Oh, Pat! What is it? What did you do?" She eagerly opened the box, and gasped. "Pat! It's *beautiful!*"

"I'm glad you like it," I said happily.

All the seasons and the times of your days...

"I *love* it. Help me put it on?"

Let the reasons and the rhymes of your days...

"Sure."

All begin and end with me...

She turned away, and I leaned over, carefully clasping the necklace before resting my hands on her delicate shoulders.

"Let me look," she wriggled off the pillows and walked over to the mirror, where she admired her new present.

We danced for the rest of the evening, easily falling into our old pattern. Carmen was still a terrific dancer after all these years. She could do it all, from Salsa to slow dancing. We always ended our evening with a slow dance.

As I held her against me, I said, "This is the way it should always be."

She looked up at me and smiled, then kissed me softly. "Always," she whispered.

For almost the next ten years, Carmen and I were solid, and our family strong. Lisa was raising Meghan close to home, Lesly went to college and then got married and had two daughters, while Laura went on to medical school. P.J. later went to college, and then followed my footsteps with a career in the import/export business. Craig went to college, too, and started looking for a future that would interest him. Carmen and I had made it through a rough patch and come through it better than ever. I truly believed that we were headed for even better times. Little did we know, however, that a tragedy was on the horizon that would change our lives forever. We were standing on the tracks and didn't see the train coming.

5

By 1996, Carmen had long been promoted into her current position at Lakeville Elementary, where she oversaw the budget for the school. In addition, she began a new business we called Creations by Carmen.

It had started when Carmen's cousin, who was getting married, had asked her for a favor. She wanted a centerpiece, and knew of Carmen's sewing prowess. Of course, she wasn't disappointed. Carmen took a ceramic swan and delicate embroidery and created a beautiful piece that became the hit of the wedding. Before she knew it, she was taking orders left and right for everything from weddings to bridal and baby showers.

"Hey hon," I said one day, trying to wedge myself in between the door and the mountains of sewing paraphernalia. Over time, Carmen had slowly turned the guest bedroom into a miniature sewing manufacturing plant. "What do you say we make you a proper space?"

"Whaddya mean?" she asked without looking up. She was working furiously on another order. I could have sworn I saw the sewing machine smoking.

"I'm gonna make you a work space." So, I hired a carpenter to build a work area in the basement that would accommodate her sewing machine, serger, and large ribbon and fabric dispensers. Next, I did all the paperwork to register her business as a sole proprietorship in Nassau County. She was then officially in business as "Creations by Carmen."

"All mine!" she exclaimed proudly, and rightfully so.

"Exactly," I replied. "And as soon as you make that first million, I'll take you public."

Carmen laughed. "You sound like Charlie Sheen in *Wall Street*. But," she put her hand over her heart. "From your mouth to God's ears, you never know."

She worked relentlessly, filling orders and creating new opportunities. I arranged for her to have a booth at a local bridal show, where she proudly hung her new sign. Things were humming along.

Then, about a year later, in 1997, she began to lose interest, declining orders and rarely visiting her workshop. When I asked about the slow down, she simply responded, "I'm really too busy at the school, and I just can't spare the time."

I thought nothing of it, but decided to keep the business name alive for a while longer, in case she changed her mind.

Later that year, I sat in my easy chair watching *The Godfather*. It was a typical Sunday afternoon, a perfect time for relaxing. Lisa passed by with a bottle of white wine and two glasses. She and Carmen were lazing about on the deck, chatting and enjoying the late afternoon.

"Is it at the part with the bloody horse head?" Lisa asked, pausing at the sliding glass door that opened onto the deck.

"What horse head?" I kidded her in mock disbelief. "*Now* you've ruined it." I'd only seen the film about 500 times.

A while passed, and then suddenly the sliding glass door flew open, rattling hard against the frame. Before I had a chance to look up, Carmen was practically on top of me. "You son of a bitch! You killed my girlfriend, Linda, and then you paid for the funeral!"

Just as I opened my mouth to speak, she threw her glass of wine in my face, and lunged for my throat. Fortunately, I was already jumping up, and grabbed her hands before she succeeded in getting her hands around my neck.

"What's the matter with you?!" I bellowed. "Have you lost your *mind*?" I would live to regret those words, but her behavior was astonishing.

"You *bastard*!" she screamed, struggling against me.

"Wha—"

"Goddamn, no good!—"

"*Carmen*! What the hell!" It was no use. Carmen just kept blasting profanities at me, trying to pull away from my grasp.

I looked over her shoulder, where Lisa stood by the open door. *I have no idea*, she mouthed.

"Lemme go!" Carmen demanded.

"You'll stop this madness?"

"Just let me go!" She pulled away, and ran upstairs. I heard the bedroom door slam closed.

Lisa and I stood there looking at each other, too stunned to speak. Finally, I wiped the wine off my face.

"What…What was that all about?" I asked Lisa.

"Dad," she said slowly. She looked about as bewildered as I felt. "I have no idea." Lisa paused, putting her hand to her forehead. "We just—we were talking, you know, about nothing. Just chatting. Then Mom said, 'I wonder what happened to my girlfriend, Linda?' I was surprised, of course. I said, 'Linda? Mom, she died four years ago in Florida. You remember. It was an asthma attack.' I was looking at her, surprised she'd forgotten, and her eyes suddenly got wild, like something just snapped."

I shook my head. *Linda was ten years ago. And why in the world would she accuse me of killing her?* It was too strange to try understanding.

Lisa continued, "And, well, you saw the rest. I'm really sorry, Dad. I didn't think it would start anything."

I put my hand up to stop her. "It's not your fault, Lisa. There's no reason for her to act like that on old news. I hadn't even talked to Linda in years before she died. It's been ten since we were together, and I wasn't in her life when she died. In fact, her family called me about a month after she died to tell me. That was it."

Neither Lisa nor I knew what to make of it, so we said our good-byes, and Lisa went home. I tiptoed upstairs to the bedroom to check on Carmen, and found her fast asleep. *I didn't think she drank that much,* I thought, puzzled.

Suddenly, I was beat. But I wasn't about to take my chances with Carmen, so I spent a restless night on the couch. I lay in 'bed' thinking, *This just isn't Carmen's style—a fiery Puerto Rican temper, sure, but violence? No.*

The next morning, I snuck into the bedroom, hoping to get into my clothes and out of the house as fast as possible.

Unfortunately, I didn't make it. As I brushed my teeth, Carmen got out of bed and started back in with the wild accusations. Jabbing her finger into my chest, she repeatedly called me every name in the book. I didn't try to defend myself or reason with her.

If I thought work would be a safe haven, I was wrong. No sooner had I walked in the door than the calls started coming in. "I'm fucking going to kill you when you get home!" If she wasn't cursing me out, she was screaming at my staff. Every time I got off the phone, another call came in. "I have a knife, you bastard, and I'm going to bury it in your chest as soon as you walk in the door!"

I called Lisa. "This is really crazy. I don't know what to do."

She thought for a moment, and then said, "I'll get her out of the house, say between six and seven. We'll go for a drive. Why don't you come home, pack some clothes, and go to a hotel—somewhere close to the office. If nothing else, it will buy us some time to sort out what is going on."

"Okay," I said, still reeling from the attacks.

That evening, I went home to pack an overnight bag. When I opened the closet to get a dress shirt for work the next day, I was stunned to find several sliced clean down the back. *She wasn't kidding about the knife.*

After checking into the Sheraton in Smithtown, I gulped a few bottles of Bud. Finally, I was able to sleep.

The next morning, with a little bit of rest, I tried again to solve the puzzle of Carmen's erratic behavior. *She is in her early fifties*, I thought. *Maybe it's her life change. Does that happen to women to this extreme? I'd better call her doctor.*

I got to the office feeling slightly better now that I had a direction. But it was upended once again when the phone rang. "It's your wife," my assistant said. "Line two."

No. No way. Not this again. I'm not going through another day of pure torture. I stared at the phone, trying to decide what to do. If I didn't pick up, she'd only call back again. And again. And again. I took a deep breath, and picked up the receiver. "Hello, Carmen," I said evenly. "What is it now?"

"Hi honey," she responded brightly. "How is your day going?"

I almost pulled the receiver away from my ear and stared at it in disbelief. *Who* was *this?* I decided to go along and see what happened. "It depends," I answered cautiously, "on what you're going to say."

"Lisa told me all about the things I did," she said. Her voice sounded back to normal, like my good old Carmen. It was sweet yet direct, entirely devoid of any hostility. "I can't remember anything."

Can't remember? Impossible! She wasn't drinking that much was she?

"I'm sorry for my actions," she continued, her voice now subdued, repentant. "It won't happen again, I promise. Please forgive me."

I wasn't buying it. The past forty-eight hours were unexplainable hell, and I wasn't going in for anymore of it. "Maybe we should activate that legal separation again, but this time," I paused a moment to make sure I meant it. "This time, carry it through to the divorce."

The gasp on the other end of the line was audible. "Divorce! Oh, please don't divorce me! Things will change, you'll see." She was crying now.

Carmen was so bare, so completely vulnerable, I couldn't help but believe her. It had to have been the wine. What else could it be?

"Okay. Okay," I said softly. I tried to reassure her. "We'll be fine. Listen, I gotta get to work now. I'll see you tonight."

She brightened again, apparently relieved that everything was back to normal. I wasn't so sure. "Can't wait to see you, honey," Carmen said. "Try to get home early and I'll make a meat loaf."

After we hung up, I phoned Lisa. "I have no idea what to say," I told her. "She needs to get checked out. Something's not right."

"Maybe. Or maybe it was the alcohol. She was drinking when I got to the house last night to get her out for a while so you could get your things. Maybe that was it. She was so upset. It's good you didn't see her. We were in my car, just driving around, and she started banging her head against the window. I tried to get her to stop, but she wouldn't. Her purse fell off her lap and I noticed there was a kitchen knife inside. I was thinking, *Oh, shit*, you know? Next thing you know, we were getting pulled over by the Nassau County Police, and I was worried he'd see the knife. But fortunately, he just asked if she's okay like that—hitting her head against the window. I told him she'd been drinking and upset 'cause you two had a fight. It was—" she paused, recollecting the incident. "It was just weird."

Weird was an understatement. I knew I couldn't sweep the last two days under the rug. I had to start looking for answers, but I realized quickly I wasn't going to get any help from Carmen, who became agitated when I mentioned the incident to her.

"Hon," I said soon after I got home. "I'm worried about you."

We were in the kitchen, where Carmen was preparing a deceptively simple and traditional Puerto Rican dish, *arroz con pollo e tostones* (chicken and rice with fried plantains). I say deceptively simple because it was simple in name only. The way she prepared each dish, adding various spices and other magical ingredients, made the food taste both succulent and complex. Carmen was a master at all her favorite foods, which reminded her of her childhood and close knit relationship with her family.

She turned briefly to look at me, and then returned to chopping up some onions. "Why are you worried?"

I took a deep breath. "Your behavior. It was...erratic. I know you don't remember, but that's just it, you don't remember."

"Oh," she waved me off. "I probably just reacted poorly to the wine. It's nothing."

"But just—could we just get you checked out?"

Immediately she slammed down the knife and wheeled on me. "Why are you *pushing* on me? I told you I'm fine. *I'm fine.*" She looked at me hard for a second, and then turned back to the cutting board. In that brief instant, I thought I saw a flash of fear in her eyes, but she turned away before I could be sure.

6

The next month or so after that was quiet, and I began to relax again. It was as if the deck incident had never happened. I'd decided to call Carmen's doctors myself. None of them, from the family physician to her gynecologist, could make any connections between Carmen's radical behavior and any possible health issues. That helped to ease my mind. I concluded that Carmen had just been tired, and the result was that her fuse was short. I began to regain my confidence that my world was back to normal for good. I couldn't have been more wrong.

Carmen and I decided that a long weekend in Puerto Rico might give us a respite from the rest of the world, and allow us to spend some time alone. Even though I was happy that things were back to normal, the strain of those forty-eight hours left me feeling frazzled. Coming so close to another separation—even worse, to a divorce—was exhausting.

We took off on a Friday, happily leaving work behind. After grabbing an American Airlines flight, we arrived in

Carmen's homeland that afternoon, got a taxi to the Caribe Hilton in San Juan, and settled in just in time for cocktails and an early dinner at the hotel. Carmen was tired after, so we turned in. It was perfect. No pressure, just pure relaxation. As I sat out on the terrace of our room and gazed out at the view, I knew that Puerto Rico's beautiful tropical landscape and rich culture was just what we needed.

We picked up relaxing the next morning, laying out by the pool for a few hours before hopping a taxi to old San Juan for some shopping. Carmen already looked tanned and rested. *As lovely as the day we met*, I thought happily, gazing at my wife's beautiful face. She wore a lightweight cream blouse and a pair of cotton shorts, and her newly manicured toes looked delicate in beige sandals.

"Let's stop in at St. Francis," Carmen suggested. It was her favorite church, and besides, the heat had already become pretty oppressive. I thought the ancient cavernous stone building would offer some relief.

"Sure, let's go."

Inside wasn't much cooler, so we said some prayers and then left. Just across the street was a small souvenir shop, so we ducked inside to cool off. The air conditioning felt good. "Let's look around a little," I said. "Then we can get some lunch."

Carmen agreed, and we started browsing. The little shop had lots of trinkets, from ashtrays and can openers to paperweights, and there were various San Juan printed t-shirts and towels hanging from the ceiling.

I left Carmen rummaging through a bin of straw hats, and headed to the back of the store to see what was there. Soon after, I heard the rising voices of two women arguing in Spanish. After a moment, I realized one of them was Carmen. I rolled my eyes. *What now?*

As I made my way to the front of the store, the voices escalated. Then Carmen came into view. She was standing face-to-face with the proprietress, a petite old Puerto Rican lady leaning against the counter.

"Whoa, whoa!" I called out, waving my arms. "What's the problema?" My Spanish had never developed over the years.

Carmen all but ignored me, while the woman behind the counter turned her head and, to switching gears into decent English, said in bewilderment, "*Señor*, this statue here is $75.00." She paused and pointed a hand carved wooden giraffe that stood about three feet tall in a display just to the right of the register. Then she drew her hand to her chest, and continued. "We negotiate all the time, but your *esposa* offer me only $5.00." She looked briefly in Carmen's direction, as if she couldn't quite grasp how anyone could make such an insult. "When I tell her no to the $5.00, she go *loca*."

At that, Carmen started to lunge over the counter. "*Loca?* I'll give you loca, you bitch!"

The old lady jumped back, and fortunately, I grabbed Carmen around the waist before she could get at her.

"Lemme go!" she yelled at me, struggling to free herself.

"Carmen! Carmen, calm down!" I yelled back, holding her tight.

As I got her feet back on the ground and steered her toward the door, I looked back at the woman. The tiny woman was pressed up against the wall, a terrified look on her face. "Sorry," I mouthed, and propelled Carmen outside.

Turning her to face me, I asked, "What's with you? I've never seen you do anything like that before."

Beads of perspiration stood on her forehead and upper lip. Her eyes were darting back-and-forth, not really focusing on anything. She was still clearly in the throes of her rage.

"Why, Carmen?" I was dumbstruck.

She thrust a finger in the direction of the store we'd just left. "*She* started it!" Carmen exclaimed. Then, under her breath, she added, "Bitch."

She's got to be joking, I thought. "It doesn't *matter* who *started* it," I said, trying to find reason in the chaos. "You're fifty-three, and she's what, ninety-five? Have a little respect."

She worked her jaw, but was silent. Then, wordlessly, she turned and marched away down the street. I paused a moment, and then went after her. When I caught up, she ignored me, focused intently on a direction unknown to me. Every few feet or so, I had to trot a little to keep pace. It must have looked comical, my six-foot two length barely keeping up with a woman a good foot shorter than him.

After searching a few seconds for an idea that might cool her off, I hit upon it. A piragua. It's basically a snow cone, but somehow totally unlike the ones you get in New York. Guys scraped the ice right off a block, put it in a cup, and then poured your choice of brightly colored syrup over it, creating a cool, super-sweet concoction. If you were really adventurous, you'd get two flavors, which would leave you in sugar shock the rest of the day.

"Hon," I reached out to touch her forearm, hoping to slow her down. "How about a piragua? Something cool."

It worked. Immediately, Carmen slowed down, and

everything about her started to relax. The intense expression on her face softened, and she looked up at me briefly. "Sure."

That was that. I was utterly confused and worried. Though thrilled to have her back to normal, I was on pins and needles wondering what might set her off again. With no small amount of trepidation, I walked beside Carmen down to the promenade where all the cruise ships docked. After getting our piraguas, we strolled along the waterfront. It was a beautiful day, despite the heat. We didn't talk much, and though I was relieved that Carmen's tension and intensity were gone, I was distracted. Ordinarily, I would enjoy a leisurely stroll, enjoying the pastel-washed stone buildings and old weather-battered military fortresses and the city wall dating back to the 16th and 17th centuries. However, I was baffled by my wife's behavior, and felt a little on edge.

A short while later, we returned to the taxi stand and got a ride back to the hotel, where we relaxed for the rest of the day. I decided not to broach the subject of the souvenir shop incident, and Carmen didn't mention it. It was as if it never happened. For the sake of the rest of the trip, I decided to keep it that way.

I made dinner reservations at one of my favorite steak and seafood restaurants, The Chart House, over on Ashford Avenue in the Condado section of San Juan. It was a Spanish colonial two-story restaurant whose second floor had a balcony that overlooked Ashford and all its activity. I knew about it from years back, when I took a local client, Pepe Llama there for dinner.

Carmen and I dressed for dinner, and then took the twenty-minute taxi ride over from our hotel, enjoying the scenery and cool breeze. Again, she looked lovely in a flowing white cotton dress with little flowers embroidered on the neckline and sleeves. I thought we made a handsome pair.

At the restaurant, we each ordered the steak and lobster tail dinner, and while we waited, Carmen sipped on a coke while I had my usual margarita on the rocks, no salt.

It was a lovely evening. We held hands across the table and made small talk. The day's events receded into the background like an afterthought. Then the food arrived. It looked great, and I was starving. I poured some A-1 on my steak, and butter on my lobster, and then picked up my knife and fork to get to work.

As I made my first cut into the steak, I noticed a 1958 Ford Fairlane passing below. Admiring its classic lines, I said, "Hey, hon, look at that car. Isn't it beautiful? You know—"

Before I could complete my sentence, I heard Carmen scream, "You son of a bitch!"

I jerked my head in her direction, only to realize she had just yelled at me.

My hands froze over my steak. "Hon, what's wrong?"

Before I could put my knife and fork down, she grabbed her plate of food and hurled it across the table at me, steak, lobster, and all landing directly on my chest. The force of the plate hitting me knocked me backward in my chair, and I hit my head on the chair of the woman sitting directly behind me before landing on the floor.

Stunned for a moment, I then scrambled to my feet as Carmen stormed out of the restaurant, and waiters hurried over to help me up. As I looked around to see what direction Carmen went, the restaurant manager arrived with a damp towel for me. I thanked him and started wiping myself off.

"I'm sorry, sir," he said, concern in his voice. "Was there a problem with the food?"

"No, no," I responded, still trying to get the food and sauces off me. "Just a problem with my wife." Still distracted, I pulled my AmEx card out. "Could I just get the check, please?"

He held his hands up, waving off my card. "Sir, it's on us. Don't worry about it."

Grateful for his kindness, I apologized for the trouble and dashed down the flight of stairs in search of Carmen.

Outside the restaurant, I looked around frantically, soon seeing her heading up Ashford Avenue. I bolted after her, and grabbed her arm. "Carmen! Hang on."

Looking for a way to diffuse the situation, I added, "I didn't like the food there, either."

She wheeled around on me and screamed, "Leave me alone!"

I looked around nervously, and it was then that I noticed two tourist police walking toward us. They'd apparently trailed me from the restaurant. I couldn't blame them. Here was this big guy chasing after a woman, and she was yelling at him to leave her alone.

One of the officers asked, "Is there a problem here, señor? They stood on either side of me, looking expectantly.

I let go of Carmen's arm. She seemed still angry, but didn't move. "No, no problem at all, thanks. My wife just had a little too much to drink," I replied, hoping to dissolve their curiosity. No such luck.

"You *bastard*," Carmen snapped. "I didn't have anything

to drink!" Then, in one sweeping move, she clocked me right in the nose with her open hand.

Immediately, my nose started to bleed, but was quickly staunched by the damp towel the manager had given me. I'd forgotten I was holding it, but was glad it came in handy.

The two police officers looked at me sympathetically, and stepped back, keeping a watchful eye on us. It was clear to them that Carmen was not being accosted.

I checked my nose, and saw that it hadn't bled much at all, and had already stopped. Before any other disaster could occur, I flagged down a cab and got Carmen inside without incident. It was a relief to see the Dos Hermanos bridge up ahead, a two hundred yard connector from which the Caribe Hilton was visible. Lights from the city sparkled on the dark water, a sight I would have enjoyed if my mind weren't occupied with getting back to the hotel.

When we got back to the hotel, Carmen walked ahead and straight to our room, all the while with me trotting to keep up and ignore the stares coming from everyone around us. I imagined they were staring at me, covered in blood, A-1 sauce, butter, and food bits.

Once in our room, Carmen went straight to the bed and lay down. Immediately, she fell asleep. I watched her for a while, not sure what to think. Then I covered her with the comforter and headed to the mini bar.

Outside on the terrace with a couple of cans of Bud, I tried to collect my thoughts and make some sort of sense out of the events of the day. *Did she want a divorce, and is acting erratically to incite me? I've heard it sometimes happens this way, but it just doesn't seem like Carmen's style. She's direct, not surreptitious.*

I was baffled, and after a few more cans of beer, I was also getting sloshed.

Just then, I heard the terrace door slide open, and Carmen stepped out. I braced myself, waiting for the worst.

"Hi hon," she said brightly. "When are we having dinner?" I'm famished."

I looked at her a moment, utterly clueless as to what to say. I figured honesty was the best policy, regardless of what reaction I'd get. "You had your dinner, Carmen, and you threw it at me." I gestured at my shirt, which I hadn't bothered to change.

She looked perplexed, and responded earnestly, "Ya know, that's not even funny. I wish you wouldn't joke with me like that."

"I'm not joking," I said firmly. "You just don't remember, and that worries me." I searched her face, looking for some clue. What should I say? What should I do?

"No," she responded, her voice cracking ever so slightly. "I don't remember, and I don't know what you're talking about."

Rather than push it, I decided to let it be. "Listen, I'm not really hungry. Why don't I just order room service? I'll get you a cheeseburger."

"Okay." She went back into the room, and I followed. "I'm going to freshen up."

How could she just drop it? I wondered. As I dialed, she went into the bathroom. I ordered the food and then sat on the bed. "Carmen," I called to her in the bathroom. "You feeling okay?"

"Yeah," she called back. "Just wiped out. I don't know, maybe it was the heat today."

"Yeah," I agreed halfheartedly. "Maybe so."

Within the hour, the cheeseburger had arrived, and Carmen had eaten half of it and a few fries. Then she was asleep again.

I went back out onto the terrace and continued working on my beers until there were no more Buds left. Then I moved on to the Heineken, and after that, a local Puerto Rican beer called "Medalla." When there was nothing left, I got up and scanned the activity four stories below. A big party was going on at an old fort called San Geronimo, with lots of flashing lights, great live Latin music, and a good sized crowd dancing away. I don't know if I was jealous of their fun or feeling sorry for myself, but at least I knew that Carmen and I should be out dancing, as well. I glanced back in the room, where Carmen was sleeping soundly, apparently utterly oblivious to both her earlier behavior and my deepening distress.

After a while, I decided we had to go home. Though we were scheduled for two more days, I couldn't chance more of the same wild behavior from Carmen. Being at home would be safer. So, I called the airline and booked us on the first flight out in the morning. I couldn't take any more chances.

7

There were no major incidents after Puerto Rico. Carmen seemed to have no recollection of what happened, and, so as not to prompt another violent outburst or upset her about what she couldn't remember, I never mentioned it. I did try again to get her to go to a doctor, but she adamantly refused. Carmen had always been a self-sufficient, strong woman. From the day I met her, she never wanted to be coddled or treated like she wasn't one hundred percent. Now was no different.

"Carmen," I pleaded, "This isn't *normal*."

"Will you leave it *alone*? Didn't you say my doctors said nothing's wrong with me?"

"No, they just said they couldn't diagnose something over the phone. They couldn't say anything's *physically* wrong. But Carmen, come *on*. It's obvious something's the matter."

"Stop fucking with me!" There was fear and anger in her voice. This wasn't Carmen, but whoever she was, this woman was not having anything to do with acknowledging something could be seriously wrong.

Not knowing what else to do, I tried to carry on with life, enjoying the Carmen I knew, and hoping the other woman would leave us alone.

The weather began to turn, and before I knew it, November was upon us. With dinner finished, Carmen took our black cocker spaniel, Rainey, out for a walk while I started clearing the table.

Rainey was a wonderful, sweet-tempered dog completely attached to Carmen, who loved her right back. Rainey came to us through Evelyn, Carmen's sister. One very rainy Saturday afternoon while driving on the Garden State Parkway in New Jersey, she noticed a dog lying in the grass on the side of the road. The poor creature was struggling to stand up, but collapsed in a heap. Evelyn realized no one else was stopping to help, and, as an animal lover, she couldn't bear to watch the dog suffer. So, she pulled over to see what she could do. Amazingly enough, the dog didn't struggle against her or lash out in pain as she negotiated getting the animal into the car.

Once at the vet's office, Evelyn learned the dog had a broken leg. On top of that, she was terribly malnourished. After setting the leg and putting a cast on it, the vet sent the dog home with Evelyn, who nursed her back to health. Evelyn searched unsuccessfully for the owners, but there were no leads. No one in the area seemed to have missed the dog, and the dog had no ID tags. When it was clear the dog had no home, Evelyn named her Rainey, appropriately enough, and later gave her to Carmen when our dog died. They were instantly attached, and took walks around the neighborhood twice a day.

Once I finished with the dishes, I went to relax in my favorite easy chair, reading the *New York Times*. After about forty-five minutes, I realized Carmen and Rainey weren't back from their walk. Neither one of them liked the cold, so to be out for almost an hour on a night like this with the temperature hovering around twenty-five degrees was unusual. If it were summer, they'd be out far longer, as Carmen liked to stop and chat with neighbors out working in their yards. That was the best time to catch up on neighborhood gossip, and both social Carmen and the personable Rainey enjoyed the conviviality.

I double-checked my watch, and then went to the front door. Just as I opened it, Rainey bounded inside, pulling Carmen along. Both were shivering from the cold, and Carmen's face was white as a sheet, her expression frozen in fear, as if she'd just seen a ghost.

Immediately, I pulled her toward me, and started rubbing her arms. "What's wrong?"

She swallowed hard, and responded, "I just had the strangest thing happen."

I reached down to unhook Rainey's leash, and then looked at Carmen expectantly.

"I couldn't find the house," her voice wavered. "And I was walking around and around looking for it." She looked at me, confused and frightened, those beautiful brown eyes begging me to help her understand.

My heart broke, but I knew I had to help Carmen. "You're okay—you must've done okay, because you're here."

"No," she shook her head. "I didn't find the house, Rainey did. I was just walking by the house now and felt Rainey's leash pull to the right so I followed her up the stairs." Carmen's eyes welled up with tears. "I was just hoping she had the right place."

She looked so vulnerable, and was so clearly shaken, I wanted to just scoop her into my arms and tell her nothing was wrong. But I couldn't do that. I didn't know what was happening, but I knew something wasn't right. I helped her out of her coat, knowing I needed to tell her something reassuring. "Hon, ya know it's windy out, and look," I pointed at her eyes. "I can see you tearing up the wind's so strong. It's no wonder you couldn't find the house with everything so blurry. Don't worry, all will be fine tomorrow."

I don't know if she believed me, but I knew I didn't.

As I lay in bed that night, I was suddenly reminded of my grandmother, May, who'd also gotten lost some fifteen years previously. My grandfather had called me at 10:30 on a Saturday morning.

"Hi Pop, what's goin' on?"

"She's not back yet. May's not back yet. She's lost." He sounded panic stricken. At eighty-years old, he was terrified.

"Slow down, Pop. Tell me what happened."

"She took the dog out, and hasn't been back for well over an hour. She *never* takes more than fifteen minutes." She took their miniature schnauzer, Max, out for walks daily, and they returned like clockwork fifteen minutes later.

"I just don't know what to do."

"Don't do anything. I'll be there in twenty minutes and I'll take a look around. Stay put in case she comes back. It'll be okay, Pop. She probably just stopped to talk to a friend."

I hung up and raced over to their apartment in Richmond

Hill, Queens, knowing it wasn't the safest place for a seventy-five year old woman to be out for a long walk. Located near the intersection of Myrtle and Hillside Avenues, it was one of the busiest intersections in Queens. Several bus lines rumbled through the area, the "J" train elevated line crossed above their back yard, and the Long Island railroad trestle snaked through all of it.

Twenty minutes later, I found a parking space about a block away from the apartment. As I headed toward the front stairs to let me grandfather know I had arrived, a police car pulled up. One of the officers got out, opened the back door, and leaned inside. May emerged from the car, bewildered and clutching little Max. The officer put his arm around her, murmuring, "It's okay, ma'am. You're home now."

I turned to address the officer, catching the frustrated look on her face. I knew she wasn't happy about something. "Officer? This is my grandmother. Is she okay?"

"She's fine, just a little shaken up. I think she walked too far and became disoriented."

I reached out to take my grandmother's elbow, and she looked up at me, her lips pursed in annoyance. "I don't understand what all the fuss is about," she protested, then looked back at the officer who'd handed her off to me. "I would have found my *own* way home."

The officer didn't seem to notice her irritation, and continued telling her story. "Your grandfather's tailor is about ten blocks from here. He saw her outside and called us. I guess he knew she was a ways from home all by herself. He gave us the address."

"Thank you, thank you," I said, making a mental note to call the tailor to thank him, too.

My grandfather was thrilled to see them. "How'd you find

them?" he asked, dropping his cane to embrace May and Max.

"I didn't," I replied, and told him what happened. The crisis was avoided.

Six years later, May passed away from complications—specifically, pneumonia—of a disease I knew little about: Alzheimer's.

I fell asleep thinking about the coincidence between May and Carmen getting lost. *Strange. Alzheimer's. That's what old people get.* It never occurred to me that the events were more than coincidental.

The next day I had an appointment with my ophthalmologist, Dr. John Brennan, for a check-up. With last night's incident, and the others piled up behind it, I knew I had to find something that explained it. Carmen's doctors hadn't made anything of them—it wasn't necessarily a menopause issue. I was wondering if maybe there was something mental going on.

I decided to mention it to Dr. Brennan. I had nothing to lose in asking what he thought, and told him the stories that had been perplexing, alarming, and saddening.

"You know," he said after listening to me. "Memory loss is not uncommon as we get older, and maybe this is happening with Carmen. Hormones do affect cognitive functions." It made some sense, but didn't explain Carmen's angry outbursts. Another was just around the corner.

8

That Sunday was our weekly food-shopping trip. Since the kids were grown and on their own, and there was just Carmen, me, and Rainey, the whole process was simplified. With great regret, I had even given up my patented aisle-by-aisle shopping note method. It made Carmen happy, at least.

Carmen agreed to let me tag along, provided I promise not to rush her through the shopping process. Of course, without my market layout, list, and troops, I was a commander without an army or the necessary weapons. Nevertheless, we bought what we needed and were back home in about an hour.

After bringing the bags in, I went straight into the living room. Like most wives, Carmen didn't want me messing with putting the groceries away. Apparently, I gave the sort of help that is a hindrance, stowing stuff away in all the wrong places, thereby driving Carmen crazy later on when she went to go find something. At this point, I didn't even bother with the appearance of helping, since that dance only resulted in Carmen shooing me out of the kitchen. Besides, I had a whole list of my own chores to do: go to the car wash, drop off and pick up clothes at the dry cleaners, stop at the Roosevelt Field Mall to buy a new briefcase, and then to Home Depot to get a power drill for Carmen so she could rebuild an old table.

I left Carmen in the kitchen, pausing a moment to watch her work. She seemed none the worse for her harrowing experience the night before with Rainey, who was now lying in the kitchen as close to Carmen as she could get without being underfoot. Good ole Rainey. "See ya, Carmen," I said, and headed out.

A few hours later, around four, I returned to the house, errands accomplished. I found Carmen in the kitchen. "Hey hon, I'm starving. How about I throw that London broil we got today on the barbeque?"

"I'm way ahead of you," she replied, turning toward me with a smile on her face. "I started marinating it in teriyaki and Worcestershire sauce about an hour ago."

I enjoyed these moments, the easy rhythms of our life together. Here was my best friend, and we were going to have a couple of steaks together, and maybe a beer or two. I smiled back as Carmen continued updating me on the food situation. "It should be ready, so why don't you fire up the grill and I'll start sautéing the mushrooms?"

"Sounds good. Do we have any of those canned white potatoes? For some reason, they go perfect with this dinner." I moved toward the cupboard without waiting for her answer.

Carmen always called the cabinet the cupboard, and I got into the habit myself. Ours was a rather tall one, about six feet high with five shelves. Carmen had to use a stepladder to get up to the higher shelves.

As I got closer, I noticed a white, creamy liquid doing a slow drip from behind the door of the bottom shelf. I opened the door, my eyes following the liquid all the way up to the top shelf. Everything was covered in it, from top to bottom. I pushed some cans and jars around before I found it: a one-gallon brick of Breyer's vanilla ice cream. The box itself had deflated when the ice cream inside melted and spilled out.

I swallowed hard, and turned around. There were only two people who could've put the ice cream there, and I never touched it. I searched around for the right way to broach the subject. "Hey, hon," I said in a jovial tone. "You musta been putting the groceries away at lightening speed."

"Yeah," she replied absentmindedly, focused as she was on sautéing the mushrooms at the stove opposite the cabinets where I was standing. "Why do you say that?"

"Well, because you put the ice cream in the cupboard instead of the freezer." I pointed over my shoulder. "See? Take a look."

She turned around and gave the open cupboard the once-over, still holding the wooden spoon in her hand. Then she exploded. "I didn't do that!" she yelled. "That's the problem with you. You blame *everything* on *me!*"

"Well, you're the one that unpacked the groceries, so I don't think Rainey here could've done it!" As soon as I said it, I felt bad. "I'm sorry, I didn't mean that."

Her face was red at this point. "You *bastard*! Why don't you ever blame those kids upstairs!"

Kids? I looked at her for a moment, trying to read her face.

Nothing but anger. "Carmen, there aren't any kids living here anymore. They were gone years ago." I was starting to feel like I had to get her to make me understand how she could say such things.

"No they're not! You go up in the attic, you'll see them," she yelled again, waving the sautéing spoon around.

"Why don't you come with me," I said quietly.

"No," she snapped, and turned back to the stove. "I have to make dinner. Don't bother me with that stuff right now."

I watched her for a while, the drying ice cream between my fingers starting to feel sticky. *I'll clean it up later*, I thought. "Yeah, Carmen, you're right. Hey, the barbeque should be hot enough now. Let's get cookin'." She didn't answer, and kept her back turned.

9

"Hey," I called, walking in the door one night. "I'm home!" The house was quiet and dark, as if no one was home. "Carmen? You home?"

"In here."

Her voice came to me from the living room. It was strangely weak and thin, as if she was straining to speak.

"What's up? You okay?" I asked, walking into the room.

"Come, sit." She patted the sofa cushion next to her.

I turned on a lamp and walked around to where she sat. At first I was going to tease her about her prim posture, but from the seriousness of her expression, I refrained. She was on the edge of the sofa, her body turned toward where she wanted me to sit.

I sat down, and she folded her hands neatly on her lap, her expression serious but a little dazed.

Reaching out to pat her hand, I asked, "Hon, what's up? You feeling alright?" At first I thought she might be having another episode, but her eyes told me I was wrong. She was too present for that.

Carmen looked at me, and then looked away, biting her bottom lip.

"Carmen?"

Finally, she said flatly, "I've got a touch of Alzheimer's."

Instantly, the blood drained from my face, and I could feel my entire body go limp. I swallowed hard, tried to speak, but couldn't. My eyes pleaded with her to tell me I heard wrong, but she kept her gaze steady, waiting for my response. Finally, I managed to speak. "Carmen," I said softly. "You can't have a 'touch' of Alzheimer's." I caught myself before my voice broke. But everything else around us had suddenly, irrevocably, shattered before our eyes.

10

Squeezing her hand, I tried to make sense of the news. *She's barely into her fifties. How can this be possible?* Suddenly, all the strangeness, all the erratic behavior of the preceding months was no longer incomprehensible. What I couldn't rationalize was how it was *possible*. Carmen, an astute, engaged, *young* woman could not have a disease that strikes people in their seventies and eighties. By comparison, Carmen was a baby.

I couldn't think past the words. I kept rewinding them over and over, and the moment I got to the point where she said, "a touch of Alzheimer's," it felt like I hit a brick wall.

There was so much to do, so much I had to find out. As I sat on the couch holding Carmen's hand, I had no idea how to start.

Carmen's quiet voice jolted me back to her, still sitting next to me. "I'm retired, now, too."

I shook my head. "Retired? The school—how does the school know?"

"It was Barbara Raber's idea for me to go to Long Island Jewish Hospital for tests."

I was dumfounded. *How could they know something was wrong and not tell me?* I was too overwhelmed for anger. That would come later. At the moment, I was trying to process what Carmen was telling me, trying to get caught up so that I could take her hand and guide her, take care of her, make everything all right again—make all this *go away*.

I reached out to touch her cheek, suddenly realizing that she had been alone in this terror. *What she must have been going through. What she knows awaits her.* "Carmen," I said gently. "You could've told me."

She smiled, pressing her cheek into my palm. Her entire face could fit in my hand. *If only we could stay just like this. I will hold her forever.*

"I didn't want you to worry," she said simply.

I shook my head. "Your worry is mine. You will never be alone in this again. I promise."

She took a deep breath, and nodded.

"Okay," I said, trying to transition into tactical mode. "We need to call the kids—wait. Lesly knows already, right?"

She nodded again. "Yes. She took me to the hospital for the tests." Seeing the look on my face, she continued. "Don't be upset with Les. I swore her to secrecy."

"Who else knows?"

"Just Lesly. I told her I wanted to be the one to tell you."

"Right, then we need to call everyone. I want to talk to Laura as soon as possible. This is—"I couldn't finish the thought. It was too overwhelming, and at that point, Carmen needed me present, strong, and ready to act. "What else did they tell you? What happens next?"

She looked suddenly exhausted. "I don't know. Lesly's got the information."

"It's okay. We'll get it all sorted out."

"I'm tired," she said. "I'm going to head up to bed."

"Do you want something to eat, first?"

"No, I'm not hungry. I just want to sleep."

I walked her upstairs, and stayed with her until she fell asleep. Then I went back to the living room, and by the light of the single lamp, called Lesly.

"Hello?"

I took a deep breath. "Hi, Les."

"Hi Dad," she said, immediately breaking down. "How could this be happening?" she pleaded through her tears. "*Especially* to Mom."

"I know," I said, my voice breaking. As the tears streamed down my face, I realized I hadn't cried in years. "We've all been dealt a bad hand, and we're going to have to pull together and help Mom."

She agreed, and we were silent for a moment, trying to grasp the reality of the situation. It was as if talking about it was making it more real than it was before. "Well," she said. "At least we have one thing in our favor."

"We do? What's that?"

"We have one of the finest treatment centers for Alzheimer's right here in our area."

"What? Where?" I felt myself reaching out to grab anything that would give us hope.

"It's the Parker Institute at Long Island Jewish Hospital. It's where I took her for her tests. I took the liberty of making an appointment this Thursday with Dr. Gisele Wolf-Klein, who is one of the directors there. We really should start treatment as soon as possible."

"I agree," I said, anxious to get started for Carmen's sake.

Though still dumbstruck by the news, at least we had a place to start. I knew already there was so much to learn, and I didn't know how to begin. I thought of the stress that Lesly must have endured, taking her mom to several appointments, not knowing what was wrong, and trying to juggle her own family at the same time. Both her girls were at an elementary school about ten miles away.

Even though Carmen wanted to tell the children herself, I knew I had to call Lisa. I just couldn't wait until Thursday to find out something—anything—about this disease.

"Lisa," I said when she answered.

"Hey there. Is everything okay?" She sounded concerned, immediately hearing the fear in my voice.

"Well, we need to talk. Can you talk now?"

"Yes, of course. Whatever you need."

I didn't know how to soften the blow, so I just came right out and said it. "Your mom's been diagnosed with Alzheimer's. We just found out today."

"Mom? Alzheimer's?" She was incredulous.

"I can't believe it. She's too young, isn't she? Could they be wrong?"

Lisa didn't speak, and I could hear she was crying.

"Lisa, come on, talk to me."

"Yeah," she managed between sobs. "Okay. I'm okay."

We spoke about our fears and worries over Carmen. Then it was time to contact Laura down in Maryland. Having finished her medical degree, she was doing her internship at the University of Maryland.

After her initial shock at the news, she put on her doctor's persona. "What do you know so far?"

"I wasn't at the hospital for the diagnosis. Carmen didn't want me to worry, so I'm really in the dark. We've got an appointment Thursday, but I can't wait. I need to know what we're dealing with here."

"It's unbelievable, Dad. But it's true, people as young as Mom can get the disease." Taking a deep breath, she continued. "The scary part is that, when that happens, Alzheimer's accelerates ten times faster than it does with someone in their seventies."

I paused to take it in, not wanting to believe it was real. "Could they be wrong? Couldn't the tests be wrong?"

"It's diagnosed on the basis of symptoms. There's no way to get in and actually see the disease. They don't…they only see it postmortem."

"So they could be wrong," I persisted.

"No," she replied quietly. "It's not likely."

We were both silent for a while. Finally, I asked, "What happens next?"

"Medication to slow the progression of the disease."

"No cure? Nothing on the horizon, even?"

"No, Dad. I'm sorry. We'll make sure Mom gets the best medicine can offer—can I talk to her?"

"She's sleeping. After she told me, everything just drained out of her. She's exhausted. I promise we'll call you tomorrow."

After we got off the phone, I made the devastating calls to the rest of the kids, all of whom were as blindsided as I was.

I was just skin and bones afterward. I barely had the energy to turn out the light, but it was better to sit in darkness than see what was coming up before my eyes.

11

That Thursday, Lesly and I took Carmen to the Parker Institute for the appointment with Dr. Wolf-Klein. We were quickly ushered into an examination room, and shortly thereafter, there was a knock on the door, and a slender woman with short ash-blonde hair entered.

Extending her hand, she said briskly but warmly, "Hello, Mr. Moffett. I'm Gisele Wolf-Klein."

Upon meeting her, I knew we were in good hands. An energetic, direct woman, Dr. Wolf-Klein was an authoritative, commanding presence. In the face of an impossible disease, she was tenacious. I was suddenly overwhelmed with a deep and new respect for people working with Alzheimer's patients and researching the disease. No longer did I feel utterly alone, but instead felt part of a vast army fighting against an enemy we had yet to understand. One thing I knew was I had a fast friend in Dr. Wolf-Klein. *Without her and her colleagues and staff,* I quickly wondered, *how will we all deal with this?*

"Let's do a quick check-up, and we'll go from there."

When she was finished, Carmen and Lesly went back to the waiting room, and I followed Dr. Wolf-Klein to her office. Once seated, I asked, "Doctor, where do we go from here?"

"First, let's go over the diagnosis. It looks like Mrs. Moffett has cognitive changes. In her condition, the most likely diagnosis would be Alzheimer's disease. How familiar are you with this disease?"

Still in disbelief, I thought, *Impossible. She's so young.* Instead, I said, "It affects people in their seventies, right?"

"Typically, yes," she said sympathetically. "But unfortunately, the disease is not exclusive to that demographic. Now, even though we cannot cure Alzheimer's, there is a lot we can do for both of you. There are medications which delay the progress, such as Aricept. And there is *support*. As a caregiver, you're going to need that." She paused to make sure I understood that the disease would affect both Carmen and me.

I swallowed, nodding hesitantly. I didn't care about me. I was grasping for the hope that drugs seemed to offer.

"So, though it's not a cure, Aricept is making its mark."

"Okay. How does Aricept work?"

"Well, it works differently with each patient. In the areas of memory and behavior, things may improve, get better in small ways, or stay the same. Things get worse, typically, over time, but the drug slows this deterioration down."

"Is there anything else I can do?"

She shook her head. Sympathetic but straightforward, I knew I was getting what I needed to know from Dr. Wolf-Klein. "Make sure she takes the medication, and keep her safe. I'd like to see her again in thirty days."

She handed me a stack of 5 mg Aricept samples, and we shook hands. Before she let go, Dr. Wolf-Klein said, "Always take care of yourself, too, Mr. Moffett. Alzheimer's can claim two victims." I nodded, but I was consumed entirely by what was ahead for Carmen.

Things could get worse, better, or stay the same, but eventually, I was going to lose my wife, my love, my best friend. I took a deep breath, and walked back to the waiting room to bring Carmen home. There was much to do to restructure both our lives, and it had to be done that very day. If I could manage that, Carmen and I could still have many good years together. After all, Alzheimer's patients didn't typically die until their seventies. Carmen was still so young.

"I'm retired. Leave me alone," Carmen said decisively.

We were sitting at the kitchen table a few days after our first appointment with Dr. Wolf-Klein at the Parker Institute. I wanted to discuss with Carmen what happens next. Where did she want to go, and what did she want to do before it was too late? What were her care directives for when the time came that she could not make decisions herself? I was pretty sure of what her answers would be to these questions, but I wanted to be clear, so that every decision I made would reflect Carmen's wishes. But she was blunt about not wanting to discuss the future.

In her mind, she was retired, and that was that. Whatever came next was simply part of the process of her life, and she didn't want to do anything differently now than she would have done had retirement come ten years later. "I just want to live my life the way I always have, and whatever happens, happens," she said.

It took me a moment to realize that part of what Carmen was saying to me was that she trusted me completely. She was, quite literally, putting her life in my hands without any doubt I would do right by her.

"Okay," I said, exhaling heavily. "You're retired."

A few days later, Carmen appeared in the kitchen with a mug. She said nothing, but simply placed it on the counter, a small determined smile flickering across her lips. Inscribed on it in bold block letters was, I'M RETIRED. LEAVE ME ALONE. I had to laugh. Leave it to Carmen to find a way to make Alzheimer's, of all things, a matter of retirement.

12

"How could you not tell me?"

I was on the phone with the Lakeville School's principal, Barbara Raber, demanding to know what had happened that led her to send Carmen to the hospital. I was so desperate to understand what had happened.

Barbara told me of a series of events that, taken together, alarmed her to the point that she thought Carmen might have some sort of mental illness. "Individually, they weren't major. Mix-ups and errors do happen. For example, there was the strange order. Airplane glue."

"Airplane glue?" I repeated, incredulous. This toxic adhesive should never be anywhere near a school, let alone in the building. As Budget Administrator, part of Carmen's job involved ordering materials and supplies for the school, as well as making up the budget for each academic year. She would have known not to order something so dangerous.

"Yes. She was supposed to order Elmer's glue. When the janitor told me he saw airplane glue in the closet, I couldn't believe it, but I figured someone down the line had made the mistake. When I asked her about it, Carmen told me she had no idea what I was talking about. Anyway, we got rid of it."

"Okay, what else?"

"There was a lost child incident. Misplaced kids had happened before, so it didn't set off any alarms for me. There was a parent who called to say she would be picking up her child, and so he shouldn't be put on the bus. Carmen had taken that call, but then didn't notify the teacher. So, the child gets put on the bus, and then the mother shows up looking for him. The problem is, no one's home, so the child goes to the neighbor's house, and they call the school. Everything worked out okay, but Carmen insisted she hadn't heard anything about not putting that child on the bus. The whole time, she was there, worrying too."

I listened intently, as Barbara told me the incident that most alarmed her.

"Three days before the yearly budget was due, Carmen was in my office, and I asked her how it was coming along, and she just gave me this blank look. Again, she told me she didn't know what I was talking about. I thought, 'Maybe she's joking.' It never occurred to me that she could be serious."

"Anything else?"

"Yes. After she left my office, I remembered I wanted to ask her something about the budget, so I went out to find her. When I asked my question, she had no recollection of the conversation we'd just had in my office. Then I knew there was no joking going on."

It was at that point that Barbara contacted the Superintendent of Schools, Sheila Terrence, and Carmen's test was ordered for the next day. Together, they contacted Lesly, who didn't want to say anything to me until after the test.

"When did all this happen?"

"Oh," she paused to think. "Over a considerable period of time."

"Give me time frames." I wanted to see if I could connect any of these episodes to the events I went through with Carmen.

"Gosh, Pat, I don't remember, exactly. Well, the budget incident, yes. But the others are just a little hazy for me. I'm sorry. And," she added quietly, "I'm sorry I didn't tell you at the time. I guess I thought you already knew, you know? I guess I just assumed Carmen would have told you about these strange events."

As I listened, I thought, *What difference does it make? Knowing won't make Carmen better.* I was grasping at straws, trying to piece everything together so I could make some sense out of it, but there was none to be made. Alzheimer's robs everyone of sense, both the patient and everyone who cares about her.

"You know, when I told Carmen she should really go see a doctor, she just sort of collapsed on herself—not literally, of course, but she just kind of wilted. Then she told me she was relieved. She'd been so scared. She said, 'Thank God, I need somebody to help me.' I suppose I knew then that she'd kept it a secret, and I thought she'd done it for a reason. "

"It's okay," I said wearily. "None of us could have known what was happening. No one thinks you get Alzheimer's in your fifties."

I hung up the phone, feeling lost and, despite what I'd just told Barbara, guilty. *Why didn't I put the pieces of the puzzle together? Why hadn't I just taken Carmen to the doctor?* In all my life, I had never felt the way I did at that moment. I failed the one I loved most. There was no consolation for that. The best I could do now was to make sure that Carmen received the very best care. I would bend over backwards to keep life for her as normal as possible, and I would walk every step of the way with her as she slowly, inevitably left me behind.

13

I quickly established a daily routine that would allow me to care for Carmen and put in a full day's work at Audiovox. I knew I had to tell my company about Carmen's diagnosis and the impact it would have on my life—and so also my work. Though I'd been with the company for twenty years, and was Vice President of International Logistics, I did not expect preferential treatment—I didn't even know what that would look like, anyway, so accustomed as I was to working long hard hours all these years. I'd never had to consider altering my work life in the profound way I was currently contemplating. At the same time, I knew I had to be honest with my employer about what I was facing, or at least what I knew at the time was before me.

Shortly after the diagnosis, I resolved to see the CEO of the company, John Shalam. Mr. Shalam had started the company from nothing back in 1964, and by the mid-1990s, had turned it into a billion dollar corporation. Throughout it all, it was a family company. Mr. Shalam always valued his employees, and we'd become a family. This was a place where people spent entire careers, so unlike the contemporary practice of job-hunting you find at many companies. When Audiovox went through tough times, as any company will, instead of laying people off, Mr. Shalam proposed a solution that saved everyone's jobs: work for less money during the rough patch, and we'd all not only keep our jobs, but we'd be compensated when the company bounced back. True to his word, there were financial rewards for everyone, and the fact that we'd been pulled together by our leader made us all that much more loyal to him. So, when I walked into his office, I knew he would do his best to help. I never expected, however, the level of support he offered.

"Pat," he said magnanimously, waving me in from behind his desk. "Come on in. Have a seat." After sitting down across from him, I told him everything I knew. "I want to keep her life as normal as possible," I said. "She deserves at least that. I know that's going to put a burden on my work life, but it's what I've got to do."

He nodded, concern etched across his face, and took in a deep breath. "Pat, I'm really sorry to hear all this bad news. And I'm sure things are going to get even more difficult as the disease progresses." He leaned forward, placing his hands on his desk. "So, let me say this. Whatever we can do for you, just let us know. If you need money, time off, or anything else that is within reach, consider it done. We're all behind you." He nodded for emphasis, a sympathetic smile briefly crossing his lips.

I swallowed hard, desperate to push down the lump in my throat. "Thanks, John. You have no idea what that means to me."

We shook hands, and I left his office, glad to be part of that organization. I couldn't think of any company that would give so much leeway under tough circumstances, and I will always be grateful for the dignified and respectful way my company treated me and my family during those difficult times.

By the time my birthday rolled around in January of 1999, a month after the diagnosis, I was feeling pretty good about managing Carmen's illness. Our routine was fairly well established. I'd get up, get breakfast ready, and depending on how Carmen was feeling, help her get ready for the day. She still took great care with her appearance, and her dress and make-up was immaculate. By the time I got home from work at the end of the day, Carmen and I were ready for dinner and then sleep. My birthday would be a nice opportunity for the family to get together and, after the initial shock and sadness of the previous weeks, have a happy occasion to celebrate.

No matter where the family was, we always tried to get together to celebrate events such as birthdays. That year was no different. Everyone agreed to assemble at the house to cut the cake, which Carmen had ordered from Carvel earlier that week. "Don't look!" she'd commanded when she brought it home earlier that day. "Not until it's time."

"Promise," I responded. "Hey, hon, while we're waiting for the kids, let's throw a couple of Porterhouse steaks on the grill before the kids arrive," I suggested. "I'll fire up the grill."

"Sounds good," she agreed. "I'm starved."

It was a typically chilly January day, but two juicy steaks were worth standing out in the cold. After about ten minutes, the grill was hot enough, and Carmen volunteered to go out with the steaks.

"I'll get to work on the salad," I offered, and started chopping up some vegetables while she put on the steaks.

Moments later, Carmen entered the kitchen holding the platter of steaks. "Here we go," she said happily. "All done."

I knew I had to do some quick thinking. The steaks were sizeable, so there was no way they'd even be seared, let alone done and ready to eat. The old me would've looked at the steaks and declared, "I can't eat a steak like that! What are you thinking?" The new me had to find a way to get them back on the grill. without upsetting Carmen.

"Hey, hon, looks great. But tell you what. I'm gonna throw 'em back on for a couple of minutes. I'm feeling like I want mine done a little more. Besides, I'm doing a hatchet job on the salad. Can we switch?"

"Sure," she responded, and handed over the platter.

I went back outside and finished the steaks, while Carmen completed the salad. Dinner went off without a hitch, and at seven, the kids arrived to cut the cake.

"Hey Dad," P.J. said, while we were waiting in the dining room for the unveiling. Carmen was in the kitchen putting the finishing touches on the cake "How does it feel to be a year older?"

Before I could answer, Carmen called from the kitchen, "So *that's* it! It's *your* birthday. Damn." The kids and I looked at each other nervously for a moment, but then Carmen entered the room holding the cake and smiling brightly. "I got to Carvel, and I couldn't remember whose birthday it was, so I told the kid to make up the top like this." She set the cake down in front of me, and stood back to admire the handiwork. "I said I'd figure it out later."

I looked down and saw the long cursive *Happy Birthday* spelled out in bright pink icing at the top arch of the cake. Beneath it was an enormous question mark.

"So, whaddya think?" She started laughing, and everyone else did, too, relieved to be able to share a moment of levity. I'd read in a book about Alzheimer's a few weeks previously that it's important to find those moments and revel in them. So long as you're laughing with the patient, the moment is a gem in the midst of great sadness and stress. As such, it is to be treasured, and we did.

I made a pot of coffee, and we finished off the cake, question mark and all. No one had a better time that night than Carmen, and I was grateful to share one last birthday with her.

14

I also decided we needed to get back to Puerto Rico before it got to the point where Carmen could no longer travel. So, I got P.J. and Craig together to plan a trip. We'd talked for years about taking such a family trip, and the boys often teased us about wanting to visit "The Motherland" where Carmen was born.

After making arrangements with our travel agent for three days at the El San Juan Hotel, with its opulent and beautiful marble and mahogany lobby and terrific ocean views from every room, the four of us boarded a plane and took the three-hour flight to the Luis Munoz Marin Airport. It would be the last time Carmen would recognize the place of her birth.

During the flight, Carmen chatted happily with our sons. Everything felt right, as if the diagnosis had been a mistake. *This*, I thought, *is how it should be.* We were a family again, one that, from all appearances, did not have a problem in the world.

After checking in at the hotel and settling into our rooms, it was almost six o'clock. We were famished, so after freshening up, we headed over to a swanky Chinese restaurant called Backstreet Hong Kong. Carmen looked stunning. There was nothing about her appearance to suggest anything was amiss. She put herself together beautifully, as she always had—of course, given her natural beauty, this was easy to do. Her look always seemed effortless. Not a hair was out of place, and her light make-up complemented the long, flowing beige skirt and white silk top.

Everything went smoothly at dinner, and we quickly fell into a routine of conversation that fitted Carmen's repetitions.

After we had ordered, Carmen commented, "I hope the waiter comes soon, because I'm starved."

"He'll be here any second," P.J. said casually.

Craig said, "It's pretty crowded tonight, so it might be a minute or two."

"Oh, okay. Well, I guess I'd better take a look at the menu."

"Good idea," I said, and handed out the menus I kept by my place setting. We didn't have to wait long before our food arrived, and by that time, Carmen had forgotten the menu sitting in front of her. She was relaxed and having a good time, and we got through dinner without incident.

Afterward, we headed toward the hotel casino. Since gambling was legal in Puerto Rico, casinos were fixtures in every hotel, which was convenient. I figured the moment Carmen got tired or disoriented, we could head back upstairs to our room.

"Boys, are you ready to lose a few quarters?"

"Actually," P.J. said, "Craig and I were hoping you two wouldn't mind if we skip the casino tonight."

"Sure, we'll manage. What's your plan for the evening?"

"It's college hoops' Sweet Sixteen. We thought we'd catch it up in our room."

"Sounds good. Mom and I will be in the casino if you want to come down later. If we're not here, we'll be back up in the room."

We said our good-byes, and Carmen and I headed into the casino. Armed with $20.00 in quarters, we sat down at two slot machines and started to plunk in coin after coin. "All right, hon," I said. "Let's try to win the mortgage—or at the very least, pay for this trip."

Carmen laughed. "I'm with you, honey. Let's go!"

After chucking a few dollars without any luck, Carmen turned to me and, smiling brightly said, "Hey, Patrick, you know what?"

"What's that hon," I said distractedly. I was trying to focus on my Lucky Sevens falling into their proper slots.

"We oughta bring the boys here some day, don't you think? They'd have so much fun."

I paused, my hand frozen on its way to grab another quarter from the bucket we'd put between us. "Yeah, hon," I said, trying to buy a second to think of a good game plan. "That's a terrific idea. But you know what?"

"What's that?" she responded, reaching in for another quarter.

"I've got a surprise for you."

"Really!" She dropped the quarter and clasped her hands together. "Tell me."

"The boys are here. They'll be down in just a few minutes."

"No, really? You're not kidding?" She beamed, clearly

pleased with this turn of events. "You know, you're just the best dad!"

I tried to shrug it off, and we played some more until Carmen got tired. Then we went upstairs to our room and went to sleep. As I drifted off, I wondered what was ahead for tomorrow.

At nine the next morning, I called over to Craig and P.J.'s room while Carmen was in the bathroom getting ready. "We're going to have breakfast on the veranda by the pool. Want to join us?"

"Sounds good," Craig said.

"Oh, and be ready for Mom to be surprised you're here." I then told them about the night before, knowing that Carmen wouldn't remember what she'd said, but would also have forgotten that the boys had come with us.

As we left our room, the boys emerged from theirs, about four doors down. Carmen saw them straightaway. "Oh my God!" she exclaimed, grabbing my arm. "Look who's here!"

P.J. and Craig turned suddenly, startled by their mother's surprise. They knew what was coming, but still looked a little stunned. It would be hard getting used to the newness of everything their mom experienced.

They waved, and walked over, keeping up the façade of a surprise trip. After hugs all around, we headed downstairs for breakfast. Carmen was delighted, and we have a wonderful reunion.

"I know," Carmen said as we finished our last cups of coffee. "Let's grab a taxi and go do Old San Juan. I can't remember the last time I was there." Carmen looked at me, as spouses usually do when one can finish the other's sentence, or fill in the details that the other can't recall. "When were we here last, Pat?"

Immediately, my mind flashed back to the terrible incident when Carmen almost jumped on top of a little old patroness at a shop across the street from St. Frances, Carmen's old church. I rubbed my head. "Jeez, hon," I said. "I don't remember. Ages ago."

"Then it's settled," she said standing up. "Let's go!"

With no small amount of trepidation, we headed over to Old San Juan, arriving in the center about eleven. We browsed at several stores without incident, and Carmen looked to be having a terrific time. We even stopped for a leisurely piragua before heading back to the hotel.

That night, we went to dinner at Ajilimojili restaurant on Ashford Avenue with P.J., Craig, and Pepe Llama and his wife, Lourdes. Pepe was an old friend and client who I always tried to see when I was in town. He and Lourdes knew about Carmen's diagnosis, and they were eager for her to have a traditional Puerto Rican meal, and Ajilimojili was the place to go. From the moment we sat down, Carmen was in her element. We literally ate everything on the menu: Sorullitos (fried corn sticks), Arañitas (fried grated plantain); Sopa de plátano (plantain soup); Chicharrones de pollo (chicken fritters); Queso frito (cheese fritters) Chorrizo (sausage); Langosta/Camarones(Lobster/Shrimp); Ensalada de Pulpo (octopus salad); Chillo Frito (red Snapper); Filete de Pescado a la Parrilla (grilled fish); Filete de Pescado Relleno (fish stuffed with shrimp/lobster).

The food just kept coming and coming, and it was delicious. The only way it could have been better is if Carmen had made it herself. Eating foods she grew up with and cooked throughout her adulthood gave her a sense of security and wellbeing, and I was thrilled she seemed so completely herself. It was as if the food had the power to help her reconnect with her identity. Unfortunately, it was short-lived.

Afterward, the four of us went to the hotel casino. This time, Carmen and I headed over to the roulette table, while P.J. and Craig sat nearby playing slot machines. Everything was going well until Carmen lost a few rounds.

"Shit!" she said suddenly. "This is bullshit!" Then she flung a few of her chips across the table and stormed off.

P.J. and Craig were already heading toward Carmen, who was striding toward the casino exit, so I gathered up her purse and our chips. To the startled onlookers, I shrugged and said, "Well, what can I tell you? The lady hates to lose." With that, I hurried off after Carmen and the boys. By the time I caught up with them in the lobby, she was chatting happily with our sons.

We left for New York the next day without further incident. As I unpacked after we got back home, I thought to myself, *Well, I accomplished what I set out to do.* The thought was bittersweet. How could Carmen and I, still so young, be making our parting plans, checking off things on a to-do list that should have been twenty years away? Still, I felt good about having that time together.

15

Before Carmen took her usual battery of tests at our next appointment with Dr. Wolf-Klein about a month later, I told Dr. Wolf-Klein how well the trip went. "There were just a couple of minor incidents—forgetting here and there—but we had a really good time."

Her eyes widened slightly as I spoke, and when I finished, she said, "Mr. Moffett, you took a big risk going on that trip."

"Really? Why do you say that?" It hadn't occurred to me that there was anything particularly risky about it, beyond a possible outburst from Carmen. I hadn't mentioned the trip to her doctor beforehand, but no one had said anything about not traveling. We were, after all, an anomaly. None of the professionals had dealt with a young Alzheimer's patient. They were used to older people who were generally homebound anyway—or who weren't going to travel very far. They just hadn't thought that we would go anywhere, and certainly, didn't know that I was the sort of guy who'd arrange a trip so far away. It was dawning on all of us that we were in uncharted territory.

"Well," Dr. Wolf-Klein explained, "Alzheimer's patients can get very agitated when in an enclosed environment like an airplane. They actually have something very much like a panic attack. It's terrible for them, and the disruption is also uncomfortable for everyone else."

"Wow," I said, taken aback. "I didn't realize it could have come to that. Carmen was so excited the whole time. She chatted away the entire plane ride with our boys."

Dr. Wolf-Klein smiled sympathetically. "I'm glad it went well, but it doesn't always. I had a case recently where a family took an Alz patient on a flight to Europe. That individual became so upset during the long flight that they had to call the rest of the trip off—and they still had to fly back here to New York!"

I reached over and patted Carmen's hand. She listened politely, seemingly unaware our conversation concerned her. "Okay, Dr. Wolf-Klein. I guess our flying vacations are over. We'll stay close to home from now on."

With that out of the way, Dr. Wolf-Klein went about the usual procedure of taking Carmen's vital signs, checking her ears, nose, and throat, and finally a blood sample. After that, we went to another room where a staff member gave her a memory test.

"Okay, Carmen," the nurse said pleasantly, sitting down across from us at a table. I'm going to show you a picture." She held up a large piece of paper with a circle drawn on it. "Now, looking at this circle, show me how you would write lines to make it look like three o'clock." She put the paper down in front of Carmen, and then slid a pen across the table.

I held my breath while Carmen peered down at the paper, studying the circle intently for some clue. Finally, she took the pen in one hand, and, holding the paper steady with the other, drew a line from the center of the circle to the area where the number 10 would be. Then she drew another line from the center to where the number 4 would be.

Relieved, I said, "Hey, Carmen, not bad! Ten to four is close to three."

The nurse smiled, "Yes, that was really good."

Carmen didn't seem bothered in the least that she couldn't get the time right, or even that she was congratulated for being close. She'd always been so sharp, and never would have tolerated anyone telling her she'd done a good job of getting an answer wrong. Still, I was thrilled she was close, and silently rooted for her throughout the test. After all, the more answers she got right, the slower the disease was progressing.

"Okay, Carmen" the nurse proceeded. "What state do you live in?"

"New York," she responded matter-of-factly.

Yesssss! I screamed silently.

"Good," the nurse said. "Now, what county do you live in?"

"Brooklyn," Carmen answered.

That's okay. At least it's geographically close to Nassau.

"Good," the nurse said again. "Who is the President of the United States?"

"Kennedy."

"What about the man sitting next to you. Do you know who that is?"

"Sure," Carmen answered without looking. "He's my husband."

I beamed. Not a great exam, but not a disaster. In a strange way, I was proud of Carmen, as if she had any control at all over what was happening to her brain.

We waited a few minutes after the exam was over, and then Dr. Wolf-Klein came in to tell us that we didn't have to come back for another appointment for four months. Without asking, I knew what it meant. Carmen's disease was progressing, and there wasn't anything anyone could do about it. Coming back for an appointment in two months wouldn't be necessary.

I patted Carmen's hand, and we stood to leave. I didn't have it in me to ask Dr. Wolf-Klein what would happen in four months.

16

"What do you say we go to Lake George?" I asked Carmen as we drove home. Lake George, in the Adirondack Mountains of upstate New York, had become our retreat years ago. We'd taken the kids there many summers, and we had many wonderful memories. As the summer of 1999 approached, I wanted to make plans for a vacation for Carmen and myself, but knew that major trips were out of the question.

"Okay," she said. "But I can't go anywhere without Rainey." I couldn't tell whether or not she recognized the name, but I knew she would have an enjoyable experience there. One thing I knew as an Alzheimer's caregiver was that you simply cannot put off what can be done right away. So, the first week of May, I called Green Mansions Townhouses to book a reservation.

Though we had stayed at a few different locations over the years, Green Mansions, just fifteen minutes north of Lake

George in Chesterton, was our favorite. The houses were located on five hundred acres, with Tripp lake on one side, a nine-hole golf course on the other, with tennis courts, and plenty of perfect places to fish and canoe.

"Yes, Mr. Moffett, you're in luck," Lynn Lewis, the office manager told me over the phone. I was worried that I wouldn't be able to get a reservation at the start of the summer season, but was relieved by Lynn's good news. "As a matter of fact," she continued, "another renter just cancelled thirty minutes ago. I hope the first week in June is okay, because I don't have anything else until mid-September."

"Yes, we'll take it," I said, pushing aside thoughts of what things might be like for Carmen in September. Alzheimer's is a living death sentence. It was just a matter of time before Carmen, for all intents and purposes, disappeared altogether. "But Lynn, I have a favor to ask."

"Sure," she said brightly. "What can I do?"

"Well," I struggled to get the words out. "Since we were last here a few years ago, my wife was stricken with Alzheimer's disease."

Lynn's gasp was audible. "Oh, Mr. Moffett, I'm so sorry. "She so young."

"Yes," I whispered, afraid speaking the words would make them real.

"Tell me, what can I do to help?"

"I was wondering if it would be okay to bring our dog, Rainey. She's a cocker spaniel, really well trained. She won't cause any trouble, really, she just sleeps all day and doesn't even bark. She—"

"Mr. Moffett," Lynn interrupted, sounding apologetic.

"You know from all the years you've spent with us that pets aren't allowed on the property."

"I know, but I hoped you could make an exception under the circumstances." My voice started to break. "This is probably Carmen's last trip."

"It's not my call," she said softly. "But I'll tell you what I can do. The townhouse you're going to rent is owned by Paul and Gloria Eike. They're a really nice couple. Let me call them and see what I can do."

I breathed a sigh of relief. "Thank you, Lynn. I don't think I can get Carmen to go without her dog."

"I'll call them and call you back."

I busied myself about the house while I waited for her call. An agonizing half hour later, the phone rang.

"Good news," Lynn said. "The Eikes said the dog is welcome. They seem to know what you're going through, and said they just want you both to have a good time."

"Thanks, Lynn. You're the best!" I was ebullient. It felt like everything was riding on our getting to bring Rainey along, and this small victory made me feel, however briefly, that some sort of progress had been made.

I had another reason to go to Lake George. Over the years, Carmen had often encouraged me to write a book about my tour in Vietnam. It was a strange experience, even as tours of duty go. I was originally scheduled to be a field grunt for the 101st Airborne Division, but through a series of coincidences and luck, that never happened. I'd told Carmen stories every once in a while over the years, and every time she'd say, "You've got to write a book. You know what they say, there is a good book in all of us. This one could be yours." I hadn't ever written a word, but I'd always had a title: *Fortunate Soldier.* Spending time at Lake George with Carmen and Rainey would give me some time to start writing. I would never have thought about sitting down to write a book, but things were different now. I could write as a triumph over tragedy in honor of Carmen.

The three weeks before our trip went by quickly, and before I knew it, Carmen, Rainey, and I were traveling on the New York Thruway in our rented Plymouth Caravan. I had it all planned out: rest stops all along the way of our three-and-a-half hour trip, even the one in Sloatsburg, only a half-hour into the trip. The kids used to goof on this when they made the journey with us. "Anyone that has to pee in Sloatsburg is a wuss!" they'd exclaim.

My only concern with stopping frequently was losing Carmen when she went into the restroom. Since I couldn't follow her in, she'd be out of my sight, and could conceivably manage to lose her way or simply remain inside. So, early on after the diagnosis, I started carrying a 5x7 laminated photograph of Carmen with me everywhere. If she went into the bathroom but didn't come out in a reasonable time, I could show my photograph to a woman about to enter, and explain that Carmen had Alz. "If you see this woman inside, her name is Carmen. Would you tell her that her husband is waiting outside?" It worked every time. Within a minute, Carmen would emerge.

We arrived at Lake George without incident, and after we checked in with Lynn, we got to our townhouse. Rainey ran circles around us as we unpacked, clearly delighted to be there. Both Carmen and I began to tire around eight that evening, so we turned in early.

The next morning, I made breakfast while Carmen sat outside on the porch enjoying the view of the lake. Rainey, thoroughly settled in, sat next to Carmen.

"Hey, hon," I called from the kitchen. "What do you say we go for a little shopping after breakfast?"

She looked over at me and smiled, the morning sun reflecting on her lovely face. "Okay."

We drove down Route 9, which fed into Canada Street, the main drag in Lake George Village. We bounced around a few shops, and then came upon a guy dressed as Frankenstein. He was trying to lure people into the House of Horrors Museum down the block.

I turned to Carmen. "Can you believe it?" I chuckled. "The guy's still at it." We'd seen the character several times over the years. "Remember how this guy would always scare the kids?"

Carmen frowned. "Kids? What kids? I don't remember any kids."

A notch in the Alz gun, I thought sadly. Every time I saw something that indicated Carmen's condition was getting worse, that's what crossed my mind.

We got back in the car and drove farther down Canada Street, passing the water slide park that the whole family always loved to visit. "Hey, hon, look!" Carmen said, her face lighting up. "Remember when Laura and Lesly used to zoom down the big slide when they first built it?"

I practically crashed into the car in front of me. I couldn't believe it. One moment she didn't remember that we had kids, and minutes later, she remembered the twins. I knew that Alzheimer's was going to do a lot of damage. Reaching over, I patted Carmen's hand. "I remember," I said.

Then I remembered something else: Minnetonka Moccasins. Two miles down the road was an Indian leather goods shop. Whenever we were at Lake George, Carmen would go to this store and find the Minnetonka Moccasins— the same ones she wore the day we met. She'd find a white pair with the beads on top, and yell across the store, "Patrick, remember these?" She never let me forget my male chauvinist remarks the day we met. In fact, she made me buy her a pair every time we were up at the lake.

The store was closed when we arrived, but I knew of another one, Indian Tepee Gifts, on Lakeshore Drive in Bolton's Landing about fifteen minutes away. We pulled up and got out of the car. "Let's go in," I suggested, taking the lead. We walked through the store together, coming upon the moccasin display. Carmen paused, and picked up a pair. She studied them intently, as if she was trying to place their significance in her life.

I waited, steps away, holding my breath.

She turned the moccasins over, her brow furrowed in concentration. Finally, she shook her head, as if to tell herself, 'no,' and then slowly returned the moccasins to their place. After hesitating a moment, she walked away.

Oh Carmen, I thought in agony. *I'm so sorry.* I was beginning to lose ground. I couldn't begin to imagine what her experience might be. From the beginning, we hadn't talked about what lay ahead. Whatever her worries were about what the slow, inexorable dissolution of her life would be like, she did not discuss them with me. Carmen had always been one to look forward, and I respected her wishes. If she was going to face this head-on, so was I.

The rest of the week went fairly well. Carmen napped or sat on the porch while I worked on *Fortunate Soldier*, amazed at how sharp my memory of conversations was. If only I could give at least some of that to Carmen.

One evening, as I wrote at the kitchen table, I looked over at Carmen, who was watching television. *It's so unfair*, I thought. *Why should I be able to call up memories from thirty years ago, and Carmen can't even remember her own children?* I couldn't write anymore that night. I put out the lights, helped Carmen into bed, and went to sleep myself. Tomorrow would be our last day, and I wanted to be sharp for the ride home.

Despite my worries, I slept well that night. There's something about the clear, chilly Adirondack air streaming through the open terrace door that put me into a deep sleep.

The next morning, I awoke feeling rested. As I gazed up at the ceiling fan, I suddenly realized Carmen wasn't in bed beside me. I sat up, listening for the television or noise in the kitchen downstairs. Nothing. I leapt out of bed and raced downstairs, calling for Carmen.

Maybe she's just gone out with Rainey, I thought hopefully. Typically, I was up and watching when Carmen would take Rainey out for morning and afternoon walks, but I had overslept. *You idiot! How could you sleep so late!* It was overcast outside, and looked like it was going to rain. *I hope she's got a coat,* I thought, casting my eyes over the gathering clouds.

Carmen and Rainey were nowhere to be found. I ran up the dirt road that separated the townhouses from the golf course, and looked around, but saw nothing. Not knowing where to go, I took off at full speed down the road past the golf course. After a half mile, I stopped. The area was deserted.

I turned back the other way, and headed toward the golf course. *She can't have gotten* that *far.*

As I ran back down the road, the rain started coming down in torrents. Off in the distance, I thought I could make out a dog on the golf course. Much to my relief, I recognized Rainey, with Carmen, dressed in shorts, a t-shirt and sneakers, holding Rainey's leash. *Oh, thank God!*

I raced up to Carmen just as the rain abated. They were already drenched. We all were. "Ah, honey," Carmen said, relief spreading across her damp face. "I'm so glad you found us. I wasn't sure of the directions back to the house."

"It's okay, it's okay," I said, putting my arm around her and taking Rainey's leash. "Don't worry, everything is fine now. It's fine." I breathed a sigh of relief, but my chest ached. I couldn't believe I'd almost lost my own wife, and that she'd been out there all alone, scared.

As the three of us walked back toward the road, soggy clothes and all, four golfers emerged from the woods to tee off. They'd been huddled under a single umbrella in the trees at the edge of the course during the rain. We were close to the road, so I didn't pay much attention to them, thinking we were almost out of the way. But then one of them yelled out, "Hey, buddy! If you're fighting with your old lady, try not to do it on a golf course where people are trying to play." I could hear a couple of them sort of snicker. It was clear to me they'd been drinking—it was never too early for a golfer to begin imbibing—or were seriously hung over.

I stopped in my tracks, and turned to face them. I couldn't believe what I'd just heard. I handed the leash to Carmen, and said, "Hon, hold Rainey for a second. I'll be right back."

As I walked toward the quartet of morons, the guy who called out to me said, "Hey, looks like the big boy's gonna kick our ass." His back-up singers laughed again. With my size, I could have done so, easily, despite the fact that I looked to have a good ten years on them, but they had clubs, and I didn't.

"Hey, assholes!" I called out. "I made a mistake today, and that mistake was sleeping thirty minutes more than I should have."

All four of them looked at me blankly, not knowing what to make of what they'd just heard.

"My wife has Alzheimer's disease, and she got out of the house without me knowing, and that was my fault. I *wish* we could fight, but we can't. Not ever again."

The bigmouth was silenced, and his friends looked away, embarrassed.

"So," I continued, "I'm not going to kick your ass when you've got a golf club in your hand, but if you really want to try me, come over to Townhouse Ten. I'll be there all morning."

As I turned to leave, one of the snicker-boys spoke up. "Hey, Mister. We were just kidding around. We didn't mean any offense."

I stopped and faced them once again. "No offense taken," I said. "But I'll tell you what. When you go home tonight and you take a shower, and dinner is waiting for you when you get out, put your arms around your wife and say, 'I love you,' because you never know when that won't matter anymore. You never know when all that's left is a ghost where your wife used to be."

Then Carmen, Rainey, and I made our way back to the house, packed up the van and headed home. I took Route 87 at Warrensburg, heading south toward New York City. About five miles later, I glanced in my side view mirror and saw the northbound exit sign: Lake George Village Exit 20. The kids got so excited when we laid eyes on that sign the first time all those years ago, eagerly anticipating the fun and adventure in store. But as the sign began to fade into the distance, I knew we would never return there again. I looked over at Carmen, who sat quietly next to me, and I began to cry helpless tears. She looked over at me and smiled, unknowing.

17

While the world anticipated the turn of the century, I sat in my house staring at the television. Dick Clark's "Rockin' New Year's Eve" show was in full swing, but I had no spirit to celebrate. The questions everyone was asking—Will computers withstand the Y2K panic? Will the stock market crash? Will planes land?—didn't matter to me. I was consumed by the blur of the past two years, and I felt lost in its haze. The future was not going to get any better.

Carmen had gone to bed at nine, and I slouched in my chair, the dark illuminated only by the flickering light emanating from the television screen. I wasn't paying attention to the show, but wanted the noise of revelers for company. When the ball dropped at midnight in Times Square and the giant "2000" sign lit up, I simply picked up the remote and turned the television off.

As the darkness enveloped me, I sat quietly listening to the distant sounds of celebration—party horns, shouts and laughter. None of that was to be for Carmen and me ever again. We used to love celebrating New Year's, happily participating in the various parties, dancing, and never-ending glasses of champagne. *Another notch.* It was then that I noticed the tears. They came easily and often in those days, sometimes without warning.

I still have a mission, I thought. *I have to keep Carmen comfortable and live as normally as possible for as long as we can.* I knew vaguely that somewhere down the road I would not be able to care for Carmen all by myself—it would become too overwhelming—and that tough decisions would have to be made. But it hurt too much to think about it, and I did not linger on the thought. I hoped that if I stayed in that darkness long enough, the thought—and the future reality it reflected—would have nowhere to land, and would simply drift away, leaving Carmen and me alone together, unharmed.

Carmen had retired from her position at the Lakeville School immediately after the diagnosis in December of 1998, but the faculty and staff had not forgotten her. She was honored the following June, along with two other retirees, at an end of the year party co-hosted by Lakeville and the Parkville Elementary School, which was located in nearby Hew Hyde Park. The party was held at Melville Hall, a distinguished old building in the U.S. Merchant Marine Academy in Kings Point. It stood in the shadow of the Throgs Neck Bridge, where the Long Island Sound feeds into the East River.

It was a lovely early evening—warm but not oppressively humid—and as I opened the car door to help Carmen out, I had to comment on how lovely she looked. She wore a long white summer dress detailed with softly colored flowers, and white pumps. She still wore her hair short, and it gently framed her heart-shaped face, and glossy red lipstick accented her lips.

"Hon, you look like a million bucks," I said. "As always."

She smiled, accepting the compliment, but something in her eyes told me she was somewhat removed from the present.

The kids were already there. Laura and Craig couldn't make it, because they were enduring their last final exams, but everyone else was there: Lesly, Lisa, Meghan, and P.J. We all sat together in a lovely room that looked out onto the river from floor to ceiling glass windows, excited to see what the school had planned. Every table had brightly colored helium balloons as centerpieces, and all the chairs were taken up by partygoers dressed for the festive, end-of-the-year event.

The two other honorees, Ana Dybner and the Assistant Principal from Lakeville, Eileen McCarthy, were retiring after many years of service to the school system. With only nine years at Lakeville, and at fifty-four years old, Carmen was the youngest honoree. And even though she'd gone on disability six months earlier, the school had not forgotten her. Everyone there wanted to wish her a farewell, and knowing it was a different sort of good-bye than what the other retirees were receiving, it was especially emotional. By formally recognizing Carmen, the school was treating her with the dignity she deserved, rather than treating her like a disabled person who leaves the building one day and is never heard from again.

The evening was fashioned after a Broadway show, and divided into two acts that consisted of various awards presentations, cocktails, appetizers, and dinner, and dancing.

We were given a program, where we saw the presentations would be styled according to *The Best of Broadway*, including *Carmen, Evita, My Fair Lady*, and *Annie Get Your Gun*. After we had cocktails and appetizers, Leslie Gussin welcomed everyone to the event. Then, it was time for Carmen's special tribute.

Almost two-dozen members of the faculty gathered at the front of the room where a stage was carved out from the ring of tables. Carmen and I sat right up front to see the performance of a song written especially for Carmen by members of the faculty club, who wore sheer black veils in the fashion of the opera, *Carmen,* and sung to the tune of "Toreador":

Carmen Moffett
Where did you go?
We're looking high.
We're looking low.
Oh, we miss you dearie, don't you know?
You should be part of the show, oh!
We miss you so-oh-oh,
We miss you so,
We miss you so-oh-oh!
Carmen Moffett
Now the time is yours!
You be the boss.
But, it's our loss.
Enjoy the many hours of the day,
Crafting and sewing away, ay!
Enjoy the day-ay-ay,
Enjoy the day,
Girl, you go all the way!

Everyone burst into applause and cheers, and Carmen laughed and clapped along. Then all the singers but two left the stage, and a solemn mood descended over the crowd. Judy Kalinowski and Sue Letosky stepped up to the podium to begin a speech they'd written in Carmen's honor.

Sue began. "Tonight we have the unique opportunity to honor Carmen Moffett, an individual I have had the privilege to work with. Carmen is a loving wife, dedicated mother and gorgeous grandmother."

Sue paused for a moment, smiling through a look of deep sadness. I reached over and squeezed Carmen's hand, and Sue continued after a deep breath to steady herself.

"As a matter of fact, she has a rather unique relationship with her sons, Patrick and Craig—some might refer to it as a mother's instinct. For example, whenever Carmen noticed either Patrick or Craig coming in the main entrance at Lakeville, she automatically opened her desk drawer, and took out her wallet before they even got a chance to say, 'Hi, Mom.'"

P.J. smiled, and nodded in agreement as Lesly, Lisa, and Meghan giggled.

"As a secretary in the Main Office, Carmen handled many tasks not stated in her job description, such as gently cleaning up a student's scraped knee or tenderly wiping away the tears from a child who had left their backpack on the school bus." These last words caught in Sue's throat, and her voice wavered. Judy leaned forward and touched her arm, and Sue paused, trying to regain her composure, but her eyes welled up with tears. She looked at Carmen, and shook her head, mouthing the word, sorry.

Carmen leaned toward me, motioning me in her direction so she could whisper in my ear. "How nice of all these people to think that much of me," she said in a tone of mild bewilderment.

I nodded my head and smiled.

Judy stepped forward, and Sue gestured for her to take over. Judy smiled at Carmen, and began. "Her warm, caring and compassionate nature was felt by colleagues, parents, students and visitors to Lakeville. Her dedication, generosity, patience and loyalty is to be greatly admired. Carmen, you have embraced us with your friendly smile and enthusiastic personality, you inspire us with your dignity and courage." Judy closed her eyes and bit her lip before regaining her composure. "Helen Keller wrote, 'The best and most beautiful things in the world cannot be seen or even touched. They must be felt with the heart.' Carmen," Judy said placing both hands over her heart, "you have truly touched our hearts." Tears streamed down her face, and her voice was barely audible as she finished. "May you be surrounded by your loving family, good friends, and God's blessing always."

There was dead silence in the room as it filled with the collective knowledge that Carmen would one day not know her friends or family anymore. Then, slowly, everyone began to clap until the sadness in the room was replaced with roaring applause. I squeezed her hand again, and wiped away my tears. There wasn't a dry eye in the room.

18

"Carmen," I said, heading toward the kitchen. "I'm famished. How bout you? When did you eat last?" It was practically time for dinner, and I suddenly realized how hungry I was. Now the question was what to make for dinner.

"October," she said matter-of-factly as she sat down on the living room sofa.

"Oh," I said, chiding myself quietly for asking the question in the first place. *Well, at least she's sitting where I can keep an eye on her. Maybe we should just order in,* I thought heading to the fridge. I was bone tired. We had some chicken breasts that I'd just bought the day before, so I thought better of calling for delivery. *I'll just put 'em on the barbeque and make some Rice-a-Roni, and that should do it.*

I pulled out the chicken and turned to the counter in time to see Carmen heading for the front door. "Hey, Carmen! Where're you going?"

"I'm going out," she replied over her shoulder.

"Oh no," I said, peeling the plastic wrapping off the package. "You can't go out now. There's too much traffic outside. We'll take a walk later."

Silence.

"Carmen?" I put the chicken down and started toward the door.

"No! I'm going out now!" Her hand was on the doorknob.

Something inside me snapped. Beginning at two in the morning, it had been a long, long day, and my brain was bent. I launched at Carmen, grabbing her around the waist before she could open the door.

As she flailed and struggled against me, I picked her up and carried her back to the sofa, where I flung her down. "Now sit the *fuck* down and don't even *think* about getting up!" I bellowed, standing over her.

A look of pure fury crossed her face. "Bullshit! You can't stop me from doing what I want to do!"

Grimacing, I shook my head. "Really? Try it again!"

She did, getting up and pushing me full force with both hands. Once again, I grabbed her around the waist and moved to deposit her back on the sofa. "You sonofabitch! Lemme go!" One of her flailing arms connected with my face, just above my left eye.

I dropped her on the sofa. It stung, and I knew there'd be a nice bruise when the night was over. Instead of fuming further, however, I took a breath. Knowing I was angry at the disease, and not at Carmen, I decided to reverse the energy. Maybe if I let her know she'd injured her man, she'd calm down. Carmen would never intentionally injure me.

Grabbing my face, I said, "Hon, stop! Don't hit me anymore. I'm hurt!"

Immediately, Carmen was on her feet. "Oh, honey, did I do that?" She put her hands on my face and drew it close to hers. "I'm so sorry. You know I would never hurt you. I love you too much for that." She put her arms around my head and held me close.

"It's okay, Carmen," I said, trying to alter the mood once again. "It was just an accident. Don't worry about it." I lifted her face to look into her eyes. "Big Irish guys like me can take a beatin'. No big deal." I winked, and she smiled, relieved everything was okay. "Now, c'mon, let's eat."

After dinner, which was without incident, we had some Jell-O while we watched our favorite evening game show line-up, *Jeopardy!* and *Wheel of Fortune*. It was our nightly ritual, with me in my favorite arm chair Carmen on the couch. Before she became ill, Carmen was always good at both games. But now, she watched in silence. I didn't know which was worse, the violence of our pre-dinner incident, or the silence that descended on the room, a silence that screamed louder than any words what Carmen was losing—and that I was losing Carmen.

Partway through *Jeopardy!*, one of Carmen's favorite categories came up. "Hey, look hon," I said, glancing over at her. "Literature."

Her expression was impassive.

Alex Trebek read the hint. "The author of this 1938 novel, *Rebecca* died in England 1989."

Before the contestants even had a chance to ring their buzzers, I heard Carmen say matter-of-factly, "Who is Daphne du Maurier?"

I practically jumped out of my chair. "Carmen!" I looked at her, then at the television, then back at Carmen. *She knows the answer! She knows the answer!* Carmen had always been an avid reader. We had books all over the house, and Carmen had read every one of them. It was astonishing that she remembered who wrote the novel, and even gave the correct response in the proper *Jeopardy!* form of a question. I was elated. I thought, *These pills really are working.*

As the show was wrapping up, I went into the kitchen for a drink. From the living room, I heard Alex Trebek signing off. "Good night, everyone," he said.

"Good night, Alex," Carmen called back.

I looked around the corner and saw her wave at the television set. It was my old Carmen, the playful woman, just being herself. For a brief few minutes that night, the world was perfect.

19

The pile of laundry in front of me looked like Mt. Everest. Though not nearly as large in reality as it was in my mind, everything felt overwhelming. I stood in our bedroom, staring at it. I'd told our housekeeper that I'd take care of folding and putting it all away, since she had a function at her child's school. Now, I almost regretted it.

With a sigh, I started folding Carmen's T-shirts. After I got a nice pile put together, I turned to her dresser and pushed down on the shirts already in the drawer to maximize space. That's when I felt something hard and bulky. I picked up the shirts and saw what looked like a Barretta lying at the bottom of the drawer. It was Carmen's old gas pellet gun. I hadn't seen it in years. *I thought we got rid of this rusty thing years ago,* I thought, picking it up. My mind drifted back to the first time I saw it, the night of the Heisman Trophy dinner in 1975.

The Holy Grail of college football, the Heisman Trophy, is bestowed on the best player of the year. It's a tremendous accomplishment to be nominated, let alone win. Nobody ever wins it more than once. Nobody except Archie Griffin. He won two years straight, in 1974 and 1975.

In those days, the Heisman was awarded annually at the Downtown Athletic Club—the DAC, as we New Yorkers called it—located in lower Manhattan just a block away from Battery Park where the Circle Line tourist boats departed for the Statue of Liberty and Ellis Island. The moment you entered the lobby of the DAC, you were greeted by the giant Heisman trophy, complete with the engraved names of all the past winners. Though the official presentation of the trophy at the DAC was mainly attended by the media, a group of VIPs, and all the nominees, the real party started about a week later at the Heisman dinner, held in the ballroom of the New York Hilton. An invitation to this party was almost as exclusive as one to the awards ceremony itself. Only three hundred guests, including many past Heisman winners like Joe Bellino, Paul Hornung, and Roger Staubach, were admitted.

After the dinner, it was customary to visit the hospitality suites on the upper floors of the hotel. These were arranged by the various ocean carriers, who would each invite their customers to a "get together" in order to pitch their services. Since I was manager of direct store imports for J.C. Penney, I was invited to all of the parties, and, as I couldn't show favoritism, I was obliged to show up to each for a drink. That didn't work out too good for me, because there were a lot of parties, and by the time I set out for the subway to Penn Station, I was hammered.

It was 12:30 am when I staggered into the station. I looked at the schedule and saw the next train on the Port Washington line, which stopped at Great Neck, would leave at 1:20. *Perfect. Now if I could just find a place to sit down and take a short snooze to sober up a bit, I'll be in good shape.* My syntax might not have been that clear, but that's about what I was thinking. I found a phone booth with a seat and collapsible doors, and immediately stuffed myself in and sat down.

No sooner had I dozed off than I was suddenly awakened by a banging on the window. I opened a bleary eye to see a nightstick with a hand attached. Upon opening the other eye, I saw the hand was attached to a police officer. "Hey, Pal!" he said through the window, pushing the doors open. "You can't use the phone booth for sleepin'. It's only for makin' calls."

"Sorry," I said groggily. "I'll leave." I started to get up, but only got halfway there before I fell back into the seat. "Whoa."

The cop peered down at me, looking over my Brooks Brothers suit. "You don't look like no run of the mill station bum," he said. "Where ya headin'?"

"Great Neck." I swallowed, my mouth suddenly dry. "On the one something train."

"Okay, that's the one-twenty train, and I'm gonna make sure you're on it.

"Thanks, offither," I slurred.

"No problem. But first, I want you to call your wife or someone that can meet you on the other end."

I closed my eyes. The only person I could call at this hour was Carmen, but she'd also be less than pleased to be awakened by a sloshed husband. *I'll make it funny,* I thought, hoping that some levity might dissolve her inevitable and justifiable annoyance. I reached up and slowly dialed home.

"Hello?" she answered sleepily on the other end.

"Hi," I started. *Not good. Try harder.* It sounded more like, 'hah.' "Lithen, I've been arrested and they're allowing me one call. I picked you."

"You idiot! What have you—"

The cop snatched the phone out of my hand before Carmen could launch into her tirade. "Gimme the damn phone," he snapped.

"Hello, ma'am?" he said in a sweet, sensible voice. "Your husband hasn't been arrested. Uh-huh, that's right. He just had a little too much to drink tonight. I'm putting him on the one-twenty. It gets into Great Neck at two. You should be there at the platform to pick him up." He eyed me as he nodded into the phone. "Uh-huh, he will. I'll see to it."

What a nice cop to go out of his way for me, I thought smiling up at him. *Carmen's nice, too. Mad at the moment, but nice.*

"I'm going to put him in the fifth car from the front, and I'll tell the conductor to throw him out at Great Neck."

Carmen must have said okay, because the cop leaned over me to hang up. I reached for the receiver, but was too late. "I was gonna tell her I love her."

"Tell her when you see her," the cop said with a hint of smile in his voice.

A few minutes later, he walked me to the train and put me on the fifth car, as promised. I think I fell asleep before I even hit the seat. The next thing I knew, the conductor was nudging me in the shoulder. "Hey, mister. This is where you get off. The officer said to make sure you got out at Great Neck."

"Thanks," I responded, my voice stronger now. The forty-minute ride felt like it had lasted only forty seconds. The sleep helped sober me up a little, so I was able to walk off the train in a fairly straight line.

The platform was empty except for a lone figure standing right in front of me, silhouetted by the dim light bulb above, hands shoved deep inside the pockets of a black raincoat with the collar up. I would have thought it was Sam Spade or a weirdo criminal but for the wool skullcap that covered short hair. White Minnetonka moccasins completed the picture and identified the person. Carmen. My Carmen.

"You look like a mugger," I said smiling.

"I *oughtta* mug you!" she yelled. Apparently, I'd not done a good job of diffusing the situation. "You ass! How could you do something like this?"

"I don't know," I said, spreading my arms. "One drink led to another, and here I am."

Wordlessly, Carmen turned away, and headed toward the car. *Even dressed like a mugger, she looks great.* Duly chastened, I followed her across South Station Road and got into the passenger side of our Chevy Malibu.

Carmen started the car, then reached into her coat pocket and tossed something onto the dashboard. It was a gun.

"What the hell is *that*?" I nodded toward the gun, recoiling a little in my seat.

"It's a gun," Carmen said, as if it was the most normal thing in the world for her to carry a gun around.

"I can see that, but why? Were you going to shoot me if I didn't get off the train?"

"It's a gas pellet gun," she explained. "I liked having some

protection when it was just me and the girls. I don't have any
pellets, but even if I did, they wouldn't penetrate *your* thick
Irish head."

She was right about that. Although the whole thing wasn't
funny at the time, it eventually became one of the family's
favorite stories.

Now, back in the present as I stood in our bedroom folding
Carmen's t-shirts, I knew I had to get rid of the gun. *If Carmen
ever got outside with this, no one would know it doesn't work...*I
didn't want to finish the thought. I put it in one of my old
sweat socks and took it out to the garbage. *What if this was a real
gun? Would my life be in jeopardy? Would Carmen accidentally
hurt me or herself? Does she think she's in danger?* Whatever her
reasons—if she even had any at this point—I didn't want to
know. I pushed the thoughts out of my mind, and finished
folding the laundry.

20

As we all know, the much-predicted disasters of the millennium never came about. There were no stock market crashes, no computer meltdowns. 2000 came and went largely without incident. Instead, the world just seemed to go about its usual chaotic business. I pressed on at work and home, trying to keep both ends burning, as Carmen's own light was slowly dimming. Daily life was a matter of pressing on and getting through.

Then, on December 28th, I got a call from the nursing home where my beloved grandfather lived. Pop was an important, deeply influential figure in my life, and I loved him dearly.

This was a man who would take a walk after work in his suit and tie, tipping his fedora to passersby as he chomped on a cigar that seemed to grow out of the side of his mouth. As he got older, he added a cane to his ensemble for support. "Keep giving in your life, and you'll be fine," he'd always told me.

"Don't ask for anything, just keep giving." He lived by those words, too.

He was the first guy in his neighborhood to get a color TV, but he hated it and simply gave it away. "That ain't color!" he declared when he turned it on for the first time. But he refused to return it. "Too much trouble, lugging that thing back to the store." So, he walked downstairs and stopped the first guy he saw on the street. "You want a color TV?" he asked the man.

"Sure," the guy answered. "But I got no money."

Pop waved him off. "I didn't ask ya if ya had money. I asked ya if ya want a brand new color TV."

"Okay, yeah."

"Can you carry it out?"

"Sure thing."

"Good. Come on up."

As the man left the building, Pop said, "And they call that color." That was Pop.

"Mr. Moffett," the nurse said. "Your grandfather has a large amount of congestion in his chest that he can't cough up. We've sent him over to Flushing Hospital to have it drained."

"Okay, what does this mean?"

"Well, other than the congestion, he's in great shape." She wasn't kidding. At ninety-eight years old, Pop was as sharp and lively as ever the last time I visited with him, and I was relieved his health was otherwise okay.

After we hung up, I bundled Carmen up and we drove over to the hospital. Other than sounding a little congested, Pop looked good. In fact, he looked no different at ninety-eight than he did in his sixties. The only things missing were his fedora and a cigar sticking out from the corner of his mouth.

He was still a big guy with an even bigger waistline, and his white hair still formed an almost perfect semi-circle from just above one ear to the other. The top of his head was shiny and smooth as a baby's bottom. As I approached his bedside, I noticed he had plenty of color, and his complaining confirmed he was feeling okay.

"Hi, Pop, how're you feelin'?" I asked.

Carmen moved to his side and reached for his hand. "Hi Papa," she said quietly.

He smiled at her and then turned to me. "Well, I'm feeling fine, Paddy, but the food stinks!" Ever the Irishman, he'd always called me Paddy.

"You ate dinner already?"

"Nah, lunch, and it was a horror."

"Well, Pop," I said smiling. "Hospital food is never gourmet."

"Yeah, I know. But this one really sucked. Anyway, let's talk about something more interesting. How's the job going?" He loved that I had a successful career. This night, to get his mind off being in the hospital, I wanted to tell him a little something out of the ordinary.

"It's going okay. I was out in the warehouse today, just passing by the receiving dock. There was this container backing in, so the clerk cuts the seal so the driver can open the doors and back in flush with the dock." Pop's eyes lit up, waiting for the punch line. Carmen sat by his side, still silently holding his hand.

"The clerk walks into the office, and I follow him in. Suddenly, there's shouting outside, 'Whoa! Whoa! Whoa!' and then a terrible crunch. So we go back outside to the dock, and underneath the truck's tires are two cases of car stereos. Completely crushed. I guess they fell out of the back of the truck and the driver didn't see them."

"Oh boy, that's too bad. But you know what, the same thing happened to me when I backed in my pickle truck one time."

"What? How? You told me you never knew how to drive, and didn't have a license. How'd you back a truck in anywhere?" I asked.

"Oh, sure, I drove. It was about 1914. I was only twelve, but in those days, everybody had to work. Anyway, I was backing my pickle truck into a warehouse on Avenue A on the lower East Side. Suddenly, one of the horses—"

"Horses!" I exclaimed. "You were driving *horses?*"

"Well, yeah. What did ya think? Anyway, one of the horses rears up and breaks one of the harnesses. Well, that was it. A barrel of pickles falls out of the back, and I ran it over."

"Well, Pop, you got me on that one."

We chatted for a while longer, and then it was time to get Carmen home and into bed. We said our good-byes, and got ready to head out. I thought about how present Pop was. Here he was, almost one-hundred years old, and could remember not only how much he hated his hospital food lunch, but also something that happened to him seventy-four years ago as if it was yesterday, while Carmen, could not remember her own name.

"Say, Paddy," Pop said as I helped Carmen put on her coat. "Do me a favor."

"Sure, Pop, what is it?" Just then, the attending physician, Dr. Patel, walked in to check Pop's chart. I introduced myself and Carmen, and then turned back to Pop.

"Here's what I want you to do. When you come by tomorrow, bring me a corned beef on rye with mustard and a knish. Oh," he snapped his finger, remembering something else. "And bring one of those pickles like we used to get on Delancy Street and a can of celray soda." He'd given me the order a hundred times, and I knew it by heart, but he loved saying the words.

As he was talking, Dr. Patel looked up, and his eyes widened. "Excuse me, Mr. Moffett," he said politely but firmly. "All those things you ordered are loaded with salt and very bad for your heart."

"Hey, doc," Pop protested. "I'm going to be ninety-nine next July, and I've eaten corned beef sandwiches all my life. So you're telling me to change my diet now so I can live to what, a hundred and two?" He shook his head. "I don't care about that, so I'm having my sandwich."

Dr. Patel sighed resignedly, and left the room. I laughed, and said, "Don't worry, Pop. I'll see you tomorrow, and I'll have everything you want to eat, just the way you like it."

"Good," he said. Then he turned to Carmen and smiled.

"I love you, Papa," she said warmly, and kissed his hand.

"I love you, too, sweetheart," he said.

I was glad she remembered him. *Heck,* I thought, *I've become grateful for all the little things.*

Carmen turned to leave, and as I moved to follow her, Pop grabbed my hand. "Hey, Paddy," he whispered. "How's she doing?"

"Slowly fading away from me, Pop. That's all I can say."

"I'm sorry, Paddy, I really am." He'd loved Carmen, and it broke his heart when I first told him about her situation.

"It's okay, Pop. I'm with her all the time, and I try to keep her spirits up." I squeezed his hand. "You get some rest, now. Sleep well."

We smiled at each other, and then I took Carmen home. It was 9:30, well past her usual bedtime these days, so I wasted no time getting her into her pajamas. She was asleep before her head hit the pillow. I watched her for a minute before turning out the light. She looked the same as ever when she slept. It was when awake that you could see something missing in her lovely eyes. I stroked her face and told her I loved her. Then I went downstairs.

Rainey and I shared a sandwich in the kitchen. It had become a habit of ours, and I was grateful for her company. "Here's the last bite," I said, handing her a piece of ham. "But I'm not sharing the wine." I decided to have a glass or two, just to relax for a while.

Carmen was the wine expert in the family. She'd even taken courses on the subject, and knew all about years and regions and brands. I was just happy if the bottle opened. Vintage was not an issue for me, but out of habit, I glanced at the year on the Pino Grigio Santa Magherita. 1998.

Moving to my favorite living room chair, I switched on the television and flipped around. Nothing was on, so I shut it off and sat in silence for a while. Though I planned to have only a glass or two, I found I had gone through the bottle easily. But for the first time in days, I started to relax a little.

After getting another bottle, I put on the Eagles' *Greatest Hits* CD. "Hotel California," "Lyin' Eyes," "Already Gone," brought back fond memories. Carmen's favorite, "Best of My

Love," started to put me in a better mood. Finally, halfway through the second bottle, I fell asleep in my recliner.

The sound of the phone woke me up. For a second, I was disoriented, but then realized I was still in my chair. *Who's calling at this hour?* I wondered, groggy from the wine and the fact that it was 5:30 in the morning.

I stumbled into the kitchen to answer the phone. "Hello?"

"Mr. Moffett?" a familiar sounding voice asked.

"Yes?"

"This is Dr. Patel at Flushing Hospital."

"Oh," I said, immediately remembering the man who'd futilely advised Pop against corned beef on rye and a knish. I was still too sleepy to be concerned about his call. "Yes, doctor, what is it?"

"I'm afraid I have some bad news." He paused for a moment before continuing. "Your grandfather passed away during the night. It had nothing to do with the congestion. It just seems that his heart gave way. I'm sorry."

I put my hand over my eyes, and lowered the receiver, automatically trying to shut out the reality of the news. After regaining my composure, I brought the receiver back up to my ear. "Thanks, doctor. I'll make...I'll make funeral arrangements and then contact the hospital."

"If you'd like an autopsy, I can arrange it."

"No, no that won't be necessary."

"All right. Again, I'm sorry."

"Thank you," I said. Then we hung up. Somehow, I made my way back to the living room and fell back in my chair. *I can't believe it. I just saw him.* I tried to wrap my mind around the words, "Pop is gone," but it didn't make any sense. One of the most important people in my life had left me. *I didn't even get him his last corned beef sandwich.*

Without thinking, I started to get up to go tell Carmen. It was instinct. But halfway out of my chair, I realized I couldn't tell her. So, I sat there alone, waiting for the dawn to break.

21

We gave Pop a nice send-off to Heaven. I was pretty confident that was his direction. Truth be told, it was Pop himself who arranged it all. All I had to do was follow his
detailed instructions. It all started with a Saturday morning
phone call years ago.

"Paddy?" It was Pop on the other end.

"Hi, Pop. How are you feeling?" From an early age, I was
always a great straight man for him.

"I'm okay. If I complained, no one would listen, anyway."

I couldn't help but chuckle.

"Listen, I need you for an hour today."

"You got it. What's up?"

"I want you to drive someplace," he said cryptically. "I'll
give you directions on the way."

Pop was always a good one for surprises, so I played along.
"All right, Pop. I'm on my way."

I drove to Richmond Hill, Queens, where I picked Pop up,

and he directed me to drive down Woodhaven Boulevard and over to Metropolitan Avenue. "Take a left here," he said, biting down on his cigar. "Then drive for about a half mile."

"Yes, Sir," I said, happy to do something nice for him.

As we approached St. John's Cemetery, Pop tapped my arm and pointed out the window. "Drive through those gates up ahead."

"Who are we visiting?" I asked. My curiosity was piqued.

"Nobody!" he responded brusquely. "Just drive."

"Okay, okay." When Pop was on a mission, I never questioned him.

After directing me to a large white building, we parked and got out. The building was quite lovely, the stone smooth and practically gleaming in the winter afternoon sun. I followed Pop inside, admiring the beautiful stained glass windows and myriad displays of brightly colored flowers.

"This way," Pop said, heading to a single elevator at the end of the marble-floored lobby. We took the lift to the second floor, and when the doors opened, all you could see were wall-to-wall, floor to ceiling crypts. Each one was marked by a gold plaque, some with inscriptions, some empty.

Pop raised his meaty finger to a crypt about four feet above the floor. "That one's mine," he said decisively. "When your grandmother and I pass on, all you'll have to do is bring us here, and they'll shove us into the wall." Typical Pop, he mimicked the movement with his own hands for good measure.

"That's a nice thought, Pop. I'm impressed." It wasn't surprising for him to organize things like this. That's just the way he operated. "This is a wonderful place to be laid to rest."

He nodded. "Now, look at all these names on the other crypts surrounding ours. Any of 'em look familiar?"

I scanned the plaques, noticing names that looked to be members of organized crime figures that died in the sixties. "Yeah, okay," I said. "So?"

"So, I planned it like this. I wanted to be around this group because May has a lot of jewelry, and nobody is gonna try to steal anything with these guys here." He smiled with satisfaction.

"Pop, not for nothin', but if someone comes to steal May's jewelry, these guys aren't gonna be much help."

With that, he burst out laughing, happy he'd pulled one over on me, or at least that he'd tried. Then he turned and, with the help of his cane, hobbled down the hall. At the end were two beautiful oak doors that opened into a large chapel. There was an altar and a half-dozen rows of satin covered folding chairs. We stood at the entrance to the chapel, taking it in. Pop said, "This is where the casket is rolled in and a small prayer service is held. After that," he clapped his hands as if wiping dirt off them. "It's over."

"Okay, Pop. I got it," I said, not wanting to dwell in the maudlin thoughts of my grandparents' deaths. "Let's go now. You're still far too alive for this place."

A few years later, my beloved grandmother passed away, and, just as Pop had arranged, so things went. It was a lovely service and burial.

Years after she'd gone, Pop brought up the subject once again while I was visiting him at the nursing home where he now lived. By this time, Carmen was ill, and I could only slip in and out to visit him before getting back home to Carmen.

"Pop, do we have to talk about this now?"

"Yes," he said firmly. "Now, listen to me carefully, Paddy."

Sitting across from him, I leaned in. "Okay, Pop. I'm listening."

"Use the same funeral home in Little Neck for me when it's my time as we did for May." He narrowed his eyes, getting ready to test me. "What's the name again?"

"Doyle B. Shaeffer," I said.

"Right, that's it. And try to use the same limo service, too. Those drivers are moonlighting cops and firemen, and they could use the money."

"Consider it done. What else?"

"I don't care what church you have the mass in, that's up to you. But," he raised his hand, "an Irish priest would be nice."

I tried to stifle a smile, but it crept around the corners of my lips. "Why don't we get twenty bagpipes to play Irish songs, too?"

He raised his eyebrows, and said in all seriousness, "Don't you think that would be a bit much?"

Laughing, I said, "Yes, I do!" Patting him on the knee, I got up. "Okay, Pop. I gotta go. Ease up off the funeral arrangements for a little while, okay? I wanna see your mug around for a few more years." I kissed him on the top of his bald head and went home. Not only did I not want to lose my Pop, I also needed to keep my focus entirely on Carmen so that I could maintain for her as normal a life as possible. But normal was over, and a call one night from Carmen's brother in-law, Tom Martinez, confirmed it.

"Hello?"

"Pat, hi. It's Tom," he said in his slow southern drawl. Tom was the husband of Carmen's sister, Millie. They lived in Manassas, Virginia, where Tom ran a small but successful construction company and Millie was a secretary at a local college. They were a solid, happy couple.

"Tom, how are ya? It's been a long time."

"Well," he said, his voice heavy. "I wish I could say I was good, but I'm not."

"What is it, Tom? What's wrong?"

He paused before answering. "It's Millie. She's been diagnosed with Alzheimer's."

At that moment, someone could have knocked me over with a feather. "What!?"

"Yup, it's true. That's the deal."

I shook my head, incredulous at what I'd just heard.

Tom continued his story. "I started to see some strange behavior in the past few months, you know, forgetting things and mood swings. At first I thought it was just hormone changes. But after I heard about Carmen, I started paying closer attention. Then we got the diagnosis."

It was astonishing. This disease had now struck two young women in the same family. Millie was only two years older than Carmen.

"I guess the doctors have told you about Aricept and Reminyl? They seem to work to slow the progress of Alzheimer's."

"Yeah," Tom said. "They did, but I refused all medication for Millie."

I almost blurted out, "What?!" again, but held my tongue.

"I think all that is just a bunch of nonsense. I'm just not going to put her through a pill regimen."

"Well, Tom, it's your call. But," I thought about what he and Millie would be in for. "As time goes on, you might want to reconsider these medications."

"We'll see. Meantime, we should make an effort to get Carmen and Millie together before it's too late, before they won't recognize each other."

"I agree," I said, and after we hung up, I called Lisa to see if she would be able to go with Carmen to Virginia. Though Carmen wasn't supposed to travel, we agreed a short flight into Dulles wouldn't hurt—and this was important.

While I stayed nervously behind in New York to work, Lisa took Carmen on a Friday morning U.S. Air shuttle to D.C., where Tom picked them up. The trip wasn't long—only through Sunday morning—it was long enough. Carmen and Millie bickered and fought from the moment they saw each other until the moment they parted. They'd always got on well, and I chalked up the fighting to the disease.

After that trip, I lost contact with Tom and Millie. It was sad, but there was no time for anything outside of Carmen. Tom and Millie were on their own.

22

By the summer of 2001, Carmen's condition had deteriorated further. Our Friday night dances, something I'd hoped would help Carmen hold on, were reduced to mere shuffles. No longer able to remember her favorite dance steps for the cha-cha, mambo, or meringue, Carmen could only make small step slow dances. When our Carlos Santana CD would play, she'd just sit down as if there was no sound in the room at all. *Oh, Carmen,* I thought, aching for her loss. How terrible she could no longer grasp what had always given her such joy—and what she had, in turn, infused with such dynamic personality. Was there anything left for her to take pleasure in? However much I mourned the slow demise of one of our traditions, I was grateful for whatever we had left. Then the day came that not only changed Carmen and I, but also the course of American history: September 11, 2001.

My attention that morning, as with all the others since Carmen's diagnosis, was on Carmen. After kissing her good-bye,

I got into my Toyota Avalon, backed out of the driveway, and got in line with other commuters heading to the Long Island Expressway.

I'd left Carmen with Craig, who was living with us at the time. Since he worked nights as a cashier at the Hammerstein ballroom, a venue for various rock bands, and didn't get home until the wee hours of the morning, he was sleeping when I left for work. With the house secured, Carmen was able to move about without constant monitoring, and I felt like everything was under control.

At just about 8:40 that morning, I muscled my way through Great Neck traffic and onto the Long Island Expressway. My usual "oldies" radio station, CBS-FM 101, was playing Gary Puckett and the Union Gap's "Woman, Woman" in the background. Back in my Vietnam days, it was one of my favorite songs. I remember, on a brief R&R to Bangkok, driving my hoochmates crazy because I played the tape over and over.

DJ, Harry Harrison, introduced Phil Pepe, a well-known New York sportswriter, with the sports report after the Union Gap finished playing. Then Harrison started spinning the Chi-Lites' "Oh Girl," one of Carmen and my favorite Friday wine night songs. But then, things got strange. Harry came on the air and said, "I've just received word now of a lot of smoke at the top of the World Trade Center—about three-quarters of the way up on Tower One. The smoke seems to be billowing out of the top. Any developments and you'll hear it right here on CBS-FM news."

Must've been some sort of accident, I thought as Harry led into Mr. G's weather report, followed by some commercials. Since the last terrorist attack in 1993 was committed using explosives four to five stories down in the garage of the Trade

Center, I figured the smoke coming from the upper stories wouldn't fit a plan to bring down the entire structure.

It was just around nine, and my forty-minute commute to Hauppauge was just halfway over. Harry closed out his show with another great oldie, "Runaround Sue," by Dion. Up to that point, it had been an almost entirely run-of-the-mill morning commute. That's when news Anchor Sue Evans came on in place of Dan Daniel, the DJ scheduled up next. "As Harry Harrison reported a few minutes ago," Evans said, "a fire was in progress at the top of the World Trade Center, we can now confirm that a jet airliner has struck the north tower. We have no information as to the airline or flight but we will get this info to you as it becomes available."

What? I couldn't believe what I'd just heard. Not believing it could have been anything but an accident, I thought, *How could a plane have hit the Trade Center on such a clear day?* My son, P.J., and I were airline buffs, so we were up to date on all the latest aviation technology. Air traffic control systems on the ground were state of the art. *This is nuts,* I thought, and called to leave a message for P.J., who I knew was in a meeting. "Hi, it's Dad. I just heard a report that a plane hit the World Trade Center. They think it was a jetliner, but it could be anything. Tell ya what though, if it's an airliner and the accident is because of traffic control problems, there's going to be hell to pay. It'll change the airline business forever. Anyway I'll call you later." I hung up, shaking my head.

As I drove on, pondering the accident, I remembered that horrible crash on a snowy day in December of 1960. I was twelve-years old when a United Airlines DC-8 collided mid-air with a TWA constellation over the Hudson River, right between the Statue of Liberty and Governor's Island. The

United jet crashed into a residential area in Brooklyn, while the constellation went down in an open field in Staten Island. 134 people died in the accident, and I remember the newspaper account of another twelve-year old boy who survived being thrown from the wreckage and landing in the hallway of a tenement house. There was also a photograph of him. His eyes were open as the doctors worked to keep him alive, but despite their best efforts, he died two hours later at a local hospital.

It was difficult reading about a kid my exact age dying. The news account was so vivid I felt like I had watched it live. The story saddened me, but at the same time, and as Pop told me, I realized I had my whole life in front of me. It was up to me to make the best of it.

Unlike that crash, however, this one occurred on a bright and clear day. It was seventy degrees and there wasn't a cloud in the sky. I concluded that air traffic control couldn't be a factor in the accident, and it didn't take long to learn I was right. I switched over to WINS news radio 1010 to see if I could learn more.

Just then, at 9:15, and with the teletype machines tapping away in the background, the reporter delivered devastating news. "We can now confirm that two jet airliners have crashed into both the North and the South towers of the World Trade Center. This is clearly an act of terrorism."

Immediately, I called P.J. again. "Son, forget my first message. We're under attack!"

After pulling into the company parking lot, I sat transfixed by the radio. A third plane had hit the Pentagon in Washington, D.C., and a fourth had crashed outside Pittsburgh. Reports were circulating about an additional eight planes still in the air, and with designated targets. At that moment, it seemed like the whole world had gone mad. Paralyzed by the shock, the whole country couldn't think of what would be coming at us next.

Suddenly, I thought, *Carmen!* I knew that everything I was hearing on the radio would also be on every television channel, which meant Carmen would be *seeing* the horror. Considering her Alzheimer's, I began to worry what effect this must be having on her. It didn't take me long to find out.

As I made my way into the building, I tried calling Carmen on my cell, but the call didn't go through. *Every cell site must be burning up with an overload of calls.* I ditched the idea of trying again from the cell, and went straight for my office.

Mary, the lobby receptionist said frantically, "Oh, Mr. Moffett, did you hear about the awful terrorist—"

"Yes, I did, Mary," I said cutting her off. "But I can't talk right now."

Dropping my briefcase on the floor of my office, I moved to pick up the phone. At that moment, it rang. Carmen. I'd set up the home phone so that my office number was on speed dial in case she needed me.

"Did you see these planes that hit those buildings?" she asked.

"Yes, I did. But everything's going to be okay, hon. Why don't you shut off the TV?"

"No," she said, and abruptly hung up.

Less than a minute later, the phone rang again. It was Carmen.

"Honey," her voice sounded vaguely nervous. "Did you know these planes hit some buildings?"

"Yes, I know. Listen to me. Craig is sleeping in the attic, and I'm going to call him. He'll stay with you today." As an afterthought I added, "He's our son. Don't worry, you'll know him when you see him." *I can't believe I just said that,* I thought with a mixture of sadness and frustration.

From another line in my office, I called Craig's cell, knowing he left it on when he was at home alone with his mom. There wasn't a landline in the attic, so I silently prayed he'd answer his cell. No such luck. The call ended up in voice mail. Meanwhile, my other line rang.

"Did you see all these people dying in those buildings?" she asked, her tone betraying her fear and shock.

"Yes, Carmen, I did. *Don't* hang up the phone, okay? Just put it on the kitchen counter."

"Okay," she said. I heard the rattle of the receiver against the counter.

At least I can keep the line open between us, I thought, putting my end of the line on speaker. Then I heard a click and realized Carmen had hung up the phone.

One of my colleagues stopped in and told me the L.I.E. had been closed to all but emergency vehicles until further notice. *Great, with companies closing up and people flooding out to the parkways, it could take me hours to get home.* The phone rang once again.

Carmen sounded really agitated. "I guess you know about these planes hitting those buildings?"

"Yes, hon," I said gently. "But don't worry, everything's going to be okay."

She seemed somewhat assuaged by my assurance, and, after saying, "I hope so," she hung up.

I've got to get to Craig. I dialed once again, and he answered. *Thank you!* "Oh, Craig, thank God I got you. Listen, planes have crashed into the Trade Center and the Pentagon. We're under attack.

"What!" he said in disbelief.

"Please, go downstairs and get Mom away from the TV. She keeps seeing the footage over and over, and every time it's terrible for her. She sees it and immediately calls me to ask if I know what's going on. You've got to get her to stop watching the news. Put on a movie or something, but keep her away from the news!"

"Okay, Dad," Craig assured me. "Don't worry. I'll take care of everything."

"Thanks, Craig. I'll call you later." With a sigh of relief, I hung up. Then I thought about what Carmen must have gone through. *She saw those planes, that terrible sight, and remembered it long enough to walk to the kitchen ten feet away and press the speed dial. After we talked for less than a minute, she probably did something in the kitchen and, by the time she got back to the living room, completely forgot what she'd seen.* With the news stations showing and endless loop of the planes hitting the towers, Carmen witnessed 9/11 as a brand new experience over and over, like repeated body blows that she could neither absorb nor anticipate. At least I, and everyone else who knew what was going on, had a baseline for the events. Shocking and terrible though it was, at least I didn't have to go through the initial shock repeatedly.

Once I collected my thoughts, I decided to figure out how to get home. P.J. and I connected, and soon were on the road. By the time we made it to Great Neck, it was late. I was too tired to cook, so I found a KFC that was still open, and got a bucket of chicken.

Carmen was glad to see us when we walked through the door, and by eight was dozing on the couch. "C'mon, hon," I said softly, helping her to her feet. "Let's get you to bed." I got her upstairs and into her pajamas, and then tucked her into bed. P.J. left shortly after for his own apartment, and Craig headed over to a friend's house.

The boys and I didn't talk about the tragedies that evening, at least not in front of Carmen. There were hushed comments here and there throughout the evening, but mostly, the three of us were deep in shock. By the end of the night, the shock slowly started being overcome by fatigue.

With the boys gone and Carmen asleep, I sat in my recliner and watched the rescue operation now underway at what used to be our dynamic Twin Towers. The devastation was beyond words. After an hour, I shut off the TV with the remote, and sat in silence. I wished I could switch off my mind, too. I didn't want to think about planes used as bombs, death all around, enormous buildings crumbling into dust, or Alzheimer's.

Eventually, I got up and put out all the lights, save for the small nightlight in the bathroom for Carmen. Thankfully my friend, Darkness, had returned briefly to rescue me once again, carrying me safely into a deep sleep. Finally, Tuesday had ended, even if September 11th never would.

23

In the wake of the 9/11 tragedy, the country began to shift from shock and disbelief to anger and deep despondency. But everyone also wanted to begin healing in the days and weeks following the terrible events. "What do we do now?" meant also "What *can* we do now?" Sadly, the same couldn't be said for Alzheimer's.

Intellectually, I knew that there was nothing I could do to help Carmen heal. But emotionally, psychologically, I was deaf to reality. You can't say to a guy who's worked in the carrier industry with some of the toughest guys in the world, a guy who's been an executive for over twenty years, a guy who's been to Vietnam—a big Irish guy from Brooklyn—that there's nothing he can do to save the love of his life. But all I could do was pray for a miracle, knowing deep inside that day would never come.

Making matters worse, Carmen's health deteriorated dramatically after 9/11. It was the equivalent of going from walking down a hill to falling off a cliff. I wondered if seeing those planes hit the buildings over and over, but thinking that each time was the first, affected her brain. Carmen's memory of the incident disappeared within seconds of turning off the television, but was there a scar, a trace left behind that pushed the disease forward? There was simply no way of knowing.

It started with calls from our neighbors, Jim and Susan, while I was at work. "Carmen's out there screaming in Spanish at the garbage men 'cause they didn't put the trash cans back where she wanted them." "Carmen's outside yelling at the gardeners. They hadn't even got out of the truck before she started." "Carmen's at the corner again with the kids." There were four small Spanish children on our block who waited on the corner across the street from our house every day with their parents for the school bus to pre-school.

"Well, Susan, what do you see her doing?" I asked, grateful Susan and Jim knew what was happening while I was away, but worried all the same about what, exactly, was going on.

"Nothing. She seems calm. The kids don't seem to mind. It's like she's watching over them. No agitation, like with the garbage guys. I get the impression of love and kindness, really."

I was relieved, and hoped the kids' parents didn't mind. I resolved to speak with them as soon as I could.

Carmen's ability to get out of the house while I was at work, and her often explosive behavior made me nervous. But the need for a caregiver was confirmed by a call from our local pizzeria. As with others in the neighborhood, I had tipped them off that Carmen's behavior might be unusual. It was our favorite pizza place, and we'd call in frequently for a pie, so, like most people in the neighborhood, they knew us well.

"Hey, Pat," I heard as I answered the phone.

"Yes," I asked, my voice tight. Calls had become cause for nervousness. "Who's this?"

"It's Coop at Napoli Pizza."

I knew right away this wasn't going to be a good call. "What's happening, Coop?"

"Nothin' serious. But you asked me to call if anything odd happened regarding Carmen."

"Yes, I did," I said bracing myself. "So, what went on?"

"We got a call from her around eleven-thirty. Baked ziti with extra sauce. She wanted to pick up, instead of having it delivered like she always did."

"So, we made up the order, but she didn't come in. Twenty minutes later, she called again. Same thing. She ordered, didn't come in. We only made up the one order. If we'd done one for every call, we'd have ten baked zitis backed up."

She never even left the house for this one. "Thanks, Coop. I'll pay you for the ziti when I get home tonight."

"No need," Coop said kindly. "It's on us." He paused for a moment, and said, "I just wish I could do more to help."

After I got off the phone with Coop, I called the sanitation company and the gardener, explaining the situation and offering to cover any extra expenses Carmen created. The next morning, I went in to work late so I could observe everything at the bus stop.

Carmen stood at the front window looking toward the bus stop. Like clockwork, as soon as the children appeared, Carmen went to the door. I noticed she had four small gift-wrapped objects in her hand.

"Hey, hon," I called after her. "Where ya goin'?"

"Just across the street," she responded. "I'll be right back."

I watched as she cross the street, gifts in hand. The children smiled and waved, and Carmen greeted the parents and hugged the children. So far, so good. After saying something to the parents, Carmen leaned over and handed each of the children a gift. There were smiles and more hugs, and then Carmen returned to the house.

The next morning when Carmen headed toward the door, I said, "Hold up, hon. I'll come with you."

She paused by the door, and then we walked across the street together. I wanted to make sure the kids' parents knew Carmen wasn't a threat to them or their children.

After saying our hellos, I pulled one of the fathers aside. "My wife loves visiting the children," I said. "Are you okay with that, or is it becoming annoying?"

"Oh, no señor," he said emphatically in heavily accented English. "She is a wonderful person, your esposa. She love children."

Relieved, I looked over at Carmen, who was watching the children open their gifts. Even though she could get agitated, I knew she'd never hurt a child. *But where'd she get presents for kids? I haven't bought any toys lately.* I turned back to the man and asked, "Señor, what kind of gifts did Carmen give the children?"

He tried to answer, but was having trouble with the words. "Zoraida," he called over to a woman. He pointed at a large nylon shopping bag she held. "She has."

Zoraida reached into the bag and took out the gifts, which I recognized right away. There was a little glass bear that was meant to clip onto a champagne glass, a porcelain swan with a bowl between its wings for holding almonds, and a small metal basket with a bow tied around it meant as a candle holder. *Carmen's inventory of wedding favors!* We still had the materials and equipment from Carmen's business, Creations by Carmen. I'd packed them away and stored them in the basement when Carmen lost interest—or what I now knew as the ability—in continuing the business.

How did she know? How could she remember where everything was, remember to wrap the little presents and then remember from one day to the next that she had them for these children? It was remarkable. An overwhelming feeling of sadness and loss descended on me as I pictured Carmen meticulously wrapping the little objects each morning for the children. *How much she must miss the Lakeville School children,* I thought.

While the experiences with the children were positive, the negatives were enough for me to realize I could no longer leave Carmen alone at any time of the day. I enlisted Craig to watch her in the morning when he could. At the time, he was studying recording studio electronics at Five Towns College, and worked nights, so his schedule was full already. Both he and P.J. would give me whatever time they could, including weekends, so I could get a little break here and there, which was greatly appreciated, but the time went by so fast that when I got back to the daily grind, I didn't feel rested at all. So, I also hired a caregiver, Olga, to stay with Carmen in the afternoons. She was a stout Russian woman born in the old Soviet Union but raised in Brighton Beach, Brooklyn,—or as we New Yorkers called it, Little Moscow, due to the heavy Russian population.

Olga, was not small in stature. I knew there would be no way for Carmen to get by her substantial frame to get out the door. On the other hand, if Carmen did get loose, she could reach Chicago by the time Olga made it to the corner. Still, the pros outweighed the cons, and on top of it all, Olga was a pleasant woman who, according to the agency that recommended her, was also highly regarded by previous clients. For the most part, things went smoothly.

We got through the Christmas holiday as well as could be expected, but it lacked the flair and warm family atmosphere that Carmen had always created. I still shopped for a tree, but the entire experience was nothing without Carmen's participation.

Every year until the kids had all grown up, the entire family would head over to Garden World in Flushing to pick out a tree amongst the thousand or so they had. The ritual was always the same. I picked up a tree from a large pile and hold it up for Carmen's approval. The kids either scampered around looking at other trees, or stood vigil next to Carmen. She'd inspect my find from a distance, and then shake her head no. In this way, we would proceed for about forty-five minutes, with the kids finally losing interest in the rest of the trees until Carmen nodded decisively, yes. The kids would erupt in cheers (and I did, too), and we'd take our treasure home.

Soon after, Carmen would turn the entire house into a veritable Christmas wonderland. She made and bought so many decorations over the years that there was not a space in the house you could look and *not* see something Christmas-y. After the house was properly decked out, she'd call the relatives over for a party. And when Carmen called, everyone, and I mean everyone came. It was as if we had the entire island of Puerto Rico at our house, ready to party.

We'd know it was going to be an especially good party as soon as we'd see family members getting out of their cars in the driveway. They'd be carrying everything from cowbells, drumsticks, and bongos, to Eddie Palmieri and Tito Puente cassettes. The best, though, was seeing Carmen's Uncle Johnny, the man who'd raised Carmen when her parents died. He would come in holding a few light green, label-less glass bottles that used to hold Bacardi but now held the festive drink, Coquito. At those times, I wished it was Christmas all year 'round. Coquito was the Puerto Rican version of eggnog—we called it Spanish eggnog. A concoction of coconut milk, egg yolks, vanilla, evaporated milk and, most importantly, one hundred proof Puerto Rican rum. Coquito was the key element to getting the party off to a flying start. Soon after it started flowing, the entire party was fired up and doing some wild salsa dancing. Once we'd worked up an appetite, we fell on the delicacies Carmen prepared. There would be pork roast, pastellas, rice and beans, and a host of her other specialties. Needless to say, Carmen's parties were legendary.

Now in 2001, the silence at Christmas was deafening, and making it through the holidays was just a chore. I couldn't bring myself to go over to Flushing for a tree. Without Carmen, it was meaningless.

With Carmen's rapid deterioration, I increased my reading about Alzheimer's, picking up as many books as I could find on the disease. I also briefly attended a caregiver's group that focused on spouses of people who were ill with Alzheimer's. But it didn't take long for me to realize my situation in that group was unique. All of them were dealing with spouses who were all over seventy. Though we could all commiserate on how horrible it is to be ill at any age, caregiving for someone with Alzheimer's at age fifty-four was far more physically demanding than someone in their seventies. I didn't go back to the support group after that first session.

As the winter slowly moved through its cycle, Carmen's disease quickly stole more of her away. In the dead of winter, Carmen forgot who I was.

We were finishing up our nightly *Jeopardy!* and *Wheel of Fortune* ritual in February of 2002. I went into the kitchen to clean up while Carmen went upstairs to the bathroom. It was close to her bedtime, so I wanted to have the house in order before winding the evening down. I walked out of the kitchen just as she was making her way back downstairs. Upon seeing me, she pulled up in mid-step. "Who are you?" she asked loudly.

"What?" Her question threw me off balance.

"Who *are* you and what are you doing here?" She sounded angry, but there was a tinge of fear underneath.

"Hon," I said smiling. "It's me, your husband."

"Oh, no," she shook her head, taking a step back up the stairs. "You're not my husband. But you better get outta here, 'cause he'll be home soon and he'll kick your ass in two seconds!"

I raised my hands. "Calm down, hon. It's me." I took a couple of steps forward. "See?"

She recoiled, shouting, "Don't you dare come near me! I'll call the police, I swear I will!"

I stopped moving toward her. "Carmen," I lowered my voice. "It's alright, it's me. Why don't you put on your pajamas and relax for a few minutes."

"You bastard!" She pointed her finger at me. *"You* don't tell *me* what to do! Now, get out of my house!"

I paused for a moment, and then decided to play along. Maybe I could temper the situation if she thought I was really leaving her house. "Okay," I said turning to leave. "I'm going now. Just don't tell your husband I was here."

She stormed back up the stairs, as I went out the front door. Outside, I took a deep breath, and figured out what to do next. After a couple of minutes, I swung open the door and loudly announced my presence. "Carmen! Honey, I'm home!"

At once, she came running down the stairs, her beautiful smile lighting up the room. "Hi honey!" She flung her arms around my neck, and planted a big kiss on me. "I thought you'd never get home!" I gave her a big hug, and guided her over to the couch. Then, even though I'd been home for hours, she asked, "So, how was your day?"

"It was okay," I said, patting her knee. "But it's late. Let's get you up to bed."

Is the day going to come, I wondered with trepidation, *when she won't ever remember me again?*

24

By the spring of 2002, I was beat. I sat slumped at my desk in Audiovox's Hauppauge corporate offices, exhausted. It wasn't the July heat that was bringing me down that day. My concerned secretary had remarked earlier about my red-rimmed eyes under which dark circles had taken up permanent residence. "You've got to find a way to give yourself a break, Mr. Moffett."

I didn't know how. Since Carmen had been diagnosed two years ago, I hadn't got a complete night's sleep, except that one night at Lake George. The consequence of that respite, losing Carmen for a terrifying half hour, was enough to keep me awake.

Even if I wasn't worried over my wife's well being, the work at home was exhausting all by itself. Carmen needed almost constant supervision. Olga, was at home with Carmen while I was at work, but the workload was still demanding—and increasingly disconcerting.

Early that morning, around two, I had awakened when I felt Carmen get out of bed. *Bathroom,* I thought, groggily. I expected her back in bed shortly, but when I heard her return, she didn't come to bed. Instead, I heard the dresser drawer open, and then fumbling around.

I opened my eyes and sat up a little, leaning on my elbow for support. With only a dim light from the hall behind her, I could just make out the silhouette of her long, pale summer nightgown. She had something in her hand, a long object, and she was taking something else—a piece of clothing?—out of the top drawer, and covering the object. Then she dropped the bundle in the drawer. It made a thud as it hit the bottom.

After she closed the drawer and returned to bed, she instantly fell asleep. though I was still heavy-headed, I decided to check it out. I got out of bed quietly and slowly opened the dresser drawer, feeling around for whatever Carmen had put in there. It wasn't long before my fingers hit on something firm. I pulled the object out of the drawer. It was wrapped up in one of Carmen's T-shirts, which I removed. It was then that I realized I was holding the handle end of our largest kitchen knife. *No, it couldn't be,* I thought in disbelief. I held it up to the backlight of the hallway, and sure enough, it was a nine-inch butcher knife. I was stunned into alertness, and suddenly my tired head started to pound.

What was she planning to do, shove it in my chest while I was sleeping? I looked over at my wife, who slept soundly just a few feet away. *Did she have a flashback of the same threat she'd made a couple of years ago about her friend, Linda?* I knew I had to do something before dawn, when Carmen would wake up.

I took the butcher knife and headed downstairs to the

kitchen, where I found the wooden block of knives on the counter—with one empty slot. I slid the knife in its place, and took the entire set downstairs to the basement. I had an old trunk in the boiler room, and I locked the knives inside. As I stood up, I shook my head. *What else have I missed?* I thought I'd covered all the bases: the gas stove dials all had child proof covers, all the exit doors had alarms on the handles, and all the windows were secure. But I hadn't thought about the knives.

I sighed, and, with heavy steps, made my way back upstairs to bed. Needless to say, I didn't sleep. I couldn't get the image of Carmen and a butcher knife out of my mind. What if I hadn't awakened to see what she was doing? Would this night, or another one in the near future, been my last on earth? Just thinking of the possibility was terrifying, and I didn't sleep the rest of the night.

The ringing of my phone brought me back to the present, and my office. I stared at it until it finally stopped, the caller sent to voice mail. I was simply too tired to speak, and decided to head home. Though only thirty miles from the office, the thought of the trip was suddenly daunting. Still, I knew if I stayed any longer, I'd become a danger on the road, both to myself and everyone else.

About two miles before my exit off the Long Island Expressway, I almost started nodding off. In an effort to stay awake, cranked up the radio until the Doobie Brothers' "China Grove" bellowed in my ears, and then switched on the air conditioner. Both hands gripping the wheel, I shook my head and yelled silently like a drill sergeant. *Come on, Moffett! Quit slacking off!* I almost smiled at the thought of myself as a slacker. If only it were true.

Once I got onto the local streets, I started to relax a little. *You're almost there.* Then, one block from the house, on Westminster Road, I saw a road crew at work in a large ditch. I slowed down, making sure to steer clear of the bright orange cones that ringed the work area, and the two workers who stood at the edge of the ditch wearing protective helmets. *Wait a sec, that's not a road worker!* It was Carmen. *Oh, Lord, what's next?*

I pulled over to the curb just ahead of the work areas and quickly got out. *Where the hell is Olga?* I thought as I moved quickly toward Carmen. "Hi, hon," I tried sounding nonchalant. "What's going on?"

She and the guy standing next to her turned toward my voice. Carmen looked perfectly relaxed, but the guy had a look that was at once both frustrated and confused.

"Nothing," Carmen replied. "Ya, know, the same old thing." Her face was glistening from perspiration, but she was beaming.

A voice called up from the ditch. "Do you know this lady?"

I peered over the edge. The other workers in the ditch had gathered around. "Yes, she's my wife. We live just around the corner." I jabbed my thumb in the direction of our house. "She has Alzheimer's disease, and wanders off sometimes. I just don't know how she got away from the caregiver," I said apologetically.

He smiled and waved off my apology. "She was just watching us work when she asked if she could wear a helmet." He shrugged. "So we gave it to her."

At that moment, Olga came lumbering up. She could barely speak, she was so winded. "Mr. Moffett! I'm so sorry."

She paused, gasping for breath. Then she wrapped a large arm across her stomach. "I had a little stomach problem and couldn't get out of the bathroom. That's when she got loose on me." She gasped again, nodding in Carmen's direction, her face covered in sweat from the heat and the exertion.

Relieved Carmen was unharmed, and grateful to the good-natured road crew, I said to Olga, "It's fine. Things are just going to happen sometimes." I turned to Carmen, reaching for her arm. "All right, hon, let's go home."

She pulled away, and retorted, "I can't go home. I'm working here!"

Oh, I hope this doesn't escalate into a major incident, I thought unhappily. It was clear Carmen really thought she was part of the crew.

"No," I shook my head. "The work day is over. See, these guys are ending the day, too." I looked over at the guy still standing next to Carmen. "Right?"

The worker's face registered understanding, and he nodded to the guys, saying, "Oh, yeah, it's quittin' time. Carmen, no more work 'til tomorrow." The rest of the guys joined in, and started climbing out of the ditch. Everyone took off their orange helmets at once, and Carmen took hers off, too.

"Okay, then," she said, handing her helmet over.

I put my arm around Carmen and started to walk toward the car. Olga was already heading back to the house, perhaps urged on by another bout of stomach upset. *It wouldn't hurt for her to lose a few pounds,* I thought fleetingly, eyeing her sizeable frame.

As I opened the door to the car for Carmen, one of the guys called out. "Hey pal!" I turned my head. "Sorry for your trouble," he said, then waved good-bye. I waved back. A small exchange that was suddenly very meaningful in the midst of our chaotic life.

"Thanks," I called back, nodding for emphasis, and got in the car.

Relieved to be back at the house, I suggested Olga go home. She didn't look well, and I figured I'd take over from here. She gratefully took up my offer.

25

There is no finer season in the finest city than autumn in New York. The combination of hearty, rustic colored leaves and the first inkling of chill in the air that renders summer's departure just a faint memory. I wanted to take advantage of this time of year to take Carmen to a Broadway show.

We had always been avid theatergoers, attending at least seven or eight shows a year at a variety of venues, including those off and off-off Broadway. In fact, we were always enthralled by the smaller theaters because we knew we'd otherwise miss wonderful performances that would likely not make it to the bigger, flashier venues.

Of course, since Carmen's illness, we hadn't been to a show. The last one was *Titanic* back in 1997 at the Lunt-Fontaine theater. At the time, the whole country was caught up in Titanic-mania. The ship had been located at the bottom of the North Atlantic, and the film of the same name was released later that year to packed theaters. Carmen and I even attended a Titanic-themed wedding (which I hoped didn't bode well for the union). The bride was so enamored of the film that she instructed the DJ to play music exclusively from the soundtrack of the film during the cocktail hour. She also had a twelve inch model of the ship at each table as the prize for some lucky attendee.

But even though it had been a long while since we'd been to see a show, I thought Carmen would enjoy, however briefly, a terrific musical. If she couldn't dance herself anymore, she might still love watching others, especially one with dancing based on the choreography of Bob Fosse. So, I got tickets in November, 2002, for a Sunday afternoon performance of *Chicago*.

I dressed Carmen in a pair of pressed jeans, cream-colored turtleneck sweater, and a pair of soft leather boots. Then, after I dressed in similar garb, I got our coats and we headed out to the city. The curtain was at 3:30, but I wanted to get us in early so we could enjoy the city before the show. To avoid the crush of theater traffic, I parked my Avalon at an indoor lot east of Fifth Avenue, and Carmen and I strolled along, window-shopping at Tiffany's, Louis Vuitton, and Saks. Then we stopped in at St. Patrick's Cathedral to light a candle. In the old days, when Carmen and I would see an evening performance, we'd sometimes make plans to stay in a hotel, attend Mass at St. Pat's the next morning, have breakfast and go home. But since Alzheimer's started running our lives, a strange, unfamiliar hotel room would only put Carmen into a panic.

After browsing along Fifth, I steered us over to Central Park. It was a perfect day. The shining sun took the edge off the cooling air, and the trees made up a kaleidoscope of vibrant colors. Reds, oranges, yellows, browns, and the last vestiges of greens spread like a canopy across the park. Carmen's eyes lit up as if seeing autumnal colors for the first time. "Oh," she sighed admiringly.

After we strolled a bit, we found a bench in a quiet area for a little breather. Carmen looked around, still taking everything in. "It's just beautiful," she said. Then she turned to me. "I don't know where I am, but thanks for bringing me here."

"It's Central Park, hon." I smiled, and put my arm around her, rubbing the back of her long camel coat to keep her warm. A chilly breeze had come up, spinning the falling leaves into little tornados.

"Is that where we are? It's changed a lot, hasn't it?"

"Yes, it has."

"It's so pretty," Carmen said, still marveling at the experience of the season's turn. "So pretty." She sat quietly for a moment, her almond eyes absorbing the scenery.

After a few minutes, I thought we'd better head back toward the theater district. Arm in arm, we made our way south on Broadway toward the 48th Street theater. As we walked along, Carmen looked up at me with a big smile and said, "I love you."

"I love you, too," I replied, patting her hand.

After checking our heavy coats, we were seated in the 10th row orchestra just five minutes before the show began. *Nice timing!* I thought, eager for every element of the afternoon to be perfect for Carmen.

From the moment the opening chords played, Carmen was rapt with attention, sometimes sitting on the edge of her seat and leaning forward to scan the stage. There was much to see in the incredibly high-energy play, which sometimes had as many as thirty dancers on the stage at a time. It was dazzling, and as I looked over at Carmen, I saw she remained utterly mesmerized by the performances.

Before I knew it, the intermission came, and I walked Carmen to the typically interminable line at the ladies' room. The line was so long, I knew I'd have time to get to the men's room and back before Carmen even made it to the door. "Hon," I touched her on the elbow. "You stay with this line, okay? I'll be right back."

"Sure," she said.

I returned in plenty of time to stand on line with her before she got to the door. "Honey," Carmen asked as we inched toward the door. "Why am I standing on this line?"

"For the bathroom."

"Oh, yeah," she nodded. "I forgot."

"That's okay. You're almost there."

As she disappeared behind the restroom door, I made a mental note of the women on line behind her. That way, if they came out and Carmen didn't, I'd know Carmen had got lost inside.

About fifteen minutes later, familiar faces started emerging from the ladies' room. *Okay*, I thought as I pulled out a 5x7 photo of Carmen. *Time to get her out.* I stopped a woman who was just walking out. "Excuse me," I said. "This is a picture of my wife. She went in about fifteen minutes ago."

The woman, who looked to be in her thirties, squinted her eyes, looking at me like I was a little off.

I quickly explained. "She has Alzheimer's disease and sometimes gets a little confused.

Immediately, her face softened, and she peered at the photograph. "What can I do to help?" she asked.

"If you could just go back into the ladies' room and find her. Just tell her that her husband is waiting for her."

The woman smiled. "Sure, I'd be glad to help. My grandma got Alzheimer's at seventy-five, so I know what you're going through."

I smiled and thanked her, thinking fleetingly to myself about the complications of the disease in an individual as young as Carmen, who was twenty-plus years younger than this woman's grandmother.

Moments later, Carmen emerged with the woman. "I found her standing in front of the mirror, but she wasn't moving at all—just standing there."

I nodded, and took Carmen's arm. "Hi honey! What are you doing here?" Carmen said, happy to see me.

"Hey," I said to the woman. "Thanks for your help. What's your name?"

"Jamie," she said.

"Well, Jamie, thanks. You rescued me today."

She smiled and said, "Glad I could help." Then she went back into the theater. Carmen and I followed suit.

If things were different, *Chicago* would have made it onto Carmen's top ten list. It was magnificent, and we both enjoyed every minute of it.

I held on tightly to Carmen's hand as we made our way through the bustling after-theater crowd. Fortunately, the crush of people didn't seem to bother her. "You know what, hon?" Carmen asked after we'd freed ourselves from the crowd and headed down Fifth Avenue.

"What's that?" I responded.

"We should really go to a Broadway show. You and I haven't done that in years."

I swallowed hard, and nodded. *Another notch.* "I'll call about tickets," I replied, my jaw set underneath a smile.

We arrived back at the parking garage, and I gave my ticket to the attendant. After a few minutes, the double horizontal doors opened, and my car emerged.

As the attendant got out, I opened the door for Carmen. "When did you get this car?" Carmen asked. "It's really beautiful."

Though I'd had it for two years, I kept it looking immaculate. "I picked it up yesterday," I said as she slid inside. "It was a surprise for you."

"Really?" she beamed. "You're so sweet!"

As I walked around to the driver's side, I caught the bewildered look on the parking attendant's face. He had been there when we'd dropped the car off, and I could see him making the connection to the woman who'd been in it just about three hours earlier. I didn't offer him an explanation, so I just gave him a tip and got in the car.

Twenty minutes later, we emerged from the midtown tunnel onto the Long Island Expressway in Queens, heading toward Great Neck. After I got Carmen out of her jeans and sweater, and into a light blouse and pants, I ordered a pizza. For the rest of the evening, we took it easy.

Around eight that night, Carmen went upstairs to wash up before bed. Suddenly, she yelled out in horror. "Hon, come quick! Come up here! There's somebody in our bedroom!"

I raced up the stairs three at a time. "Who's here?" I asked, racing into the bedroom.

Carmen was frozen in front of the mirror, her beautiful face frozen in terror. Her hand shaking, she pointed at her reflection. "Right there, see?" she said, her voice quivering.

It must be horrible to become a stranger to yourself. Immediately, I turned everything down to calm, remembering reading recently about this very phenomenon. Called misidentification, the phenomenon is terrifying to the individual going through it. "Carmen, it's okay," I said, moving to put my arm around her. "That's you. See, look at how it's the both of us together."

"No!" she cried, pushing against me. "No, it isn't. Don't argue with me!" Then she went into full panic mode. "Damn it! Why can't you agree with *anything* I say! I *hate you!*"

"You don't hate me," I said as I pulled her away from the mirror. I knew I had to get her mind off the threatening reflection. "Just calm down."

"Get the fuck away from me!" she screamed, fighting against my grasp. "I don't need you anymore, so just get *out* of this room!"

I released her, and moved out of range of her flailing fists. "Okay, Carmen. Okay. I'll be downstairs if you need me. Okay?"

"Drop dead," she replied, turning away from me.

From my recliner in the living room, I could hear her upstairs pacing non-stop from room to room. I half-watched the television, waiting for Carmen to calm down. Eventually, the pacing stopped, and I went upstairs to check on her. I found her fast asleep, fully clothed, on the bed.

"Carmen," I whispered softly. "Let's get you into your pajamas."

Still mostly asleep, she got up into a sitting position, but as soon as I went to unbutton her blouse, she started swinging. I kept ducking, but eventually knew it was no use. Taking a few steps back, I waited for Carmen to lie back down. Then I covered her with the comforter, and let her sleep. *It's okay,* I told myself. *The day was still good.* I was glad we were able to share our last Broadway show together. I knew there would be no more.

26

The coming months saw Carmen's agitation intensify. The moment I would walk in the door, she'd start yelling at me. One look at Olga would tell me it had been a trying day. The violence only increased, and one day, Olga told me she was almost at her end. "It was a long, tough day, Mr. Moffett," she said apologetically. "I'm not sure how much longer I can go on."

I couldn't blame her. Carmen just couldn't settle down for more than two minutes at a time. She roamed the house constantly, and Olga had a difficult time keeping up with her. On top of that, she often got physical with Laudi, our housekeeper.

Laudi came in for a half day once a week to help me keep on top of the cleaning. "Mr. Patrick," she said the day she quit, "I no come no more." She looked both sad and frightened. "Miss Carmen, she hit me all the time I work."

"I'm sorry," I said, knowing there was nothing I could do to keep Laudi safe. I was sad to lose her, but, as with Olga, I couldn't blame her.

"I know Miss Carmen is mucho inferma," Laudi continued. "But I can help no more."

"Don't worry. You did your best, and I appreciate everything you did for us." It was true. Laudi had worked around Carmen's attacks for some time. Some were simply annoyances, such as when Carmen would hit Laudi with pillows while she was making the bed, or throw fresh laundry around the room after Laudi had carefully folded it. The turning point, however, was when Carmen started smacking her. Understandably, Laudi was both hurt and frightened.

After Laudi quit, and with time running out on Olga, I knew I had to reorganize. I took time off from work so I could be with Carmen more every day. It was important to keep everything as routine as possible. We even attended five o'clock mass at St. Aloysius Church, which Carmen loved. But problems would get worse when the sun went down. Carmen was much more violent at night than she was during the day, and in vain I searched for what set her off each time. The only constant I could find with the violence was darkness, and I searched my Alzheimer's guidebooks for any known behavior similar to what Carmen experienced. *There it is. "Sundowning."*

A behavioral disorder in Alzheimer's patients, sundowning manifests itself at the end of the day and into the evening, and is thought to be associated with poor sleep quality and simply being tired. *Well, at least there's a name for it*, I thought. But I had no idea how to mitigate the behavior, both for Carmen's sake as well as my own. For a petite, otherwise remarkably gentle woman to become as physically hostile as Carmen did at night was something of a shock to me. I was supposed to be able to handle anything.

It wasn't long before daytime wasn't that much better. Olga spent a good part of her day ducking Carmen's fists, and the result was inevitable. "Mr. Moffett," she told me, shaking her head. "I've got to give you my notice. I just can't handle Carmen anymore. I feel like I'm in danger every day."

"I know, Olga," I said. "It's okay, I understand." Carmen's outbursts with Olga were on the same order as what happened with Laudi. Carmen might throw a freshly made sandwich at her, or upend a checkerboard and toss it at her while they would play a game. It was the direct physical attacks, however, that pushed Olga over the edge.

"I will stay until you can find a replacement," she offered.

There isn't going to be any replacement, I thought. *That would be like finding a sparring partner for Muhammad Ali.* "No, that's okay, Olga. Just stay with me until I can make arrangements at a daycare center full time. I knew it was time to call the Long Island Jewish Hospital's Granat Center.

27

Located at the Parker Jewish Institute, the Granat Center opened in August, 1989 through a grant from the Robert Wood Johnson Foundation. It was Dr. Wolf-Klein, Carmen's Alzheimer's specialist and world-renown geriatrician, who wrote the original grant. Since its inception, the Granat Center has offered day care services for persons with Alzheimer's disease and related dementias. In fact, at least through the time this book was first published, Granat's social day care model was the only such one for dementia care and respite services in downstate New York. Designed specifically to provide much needed respite for the caregiver from the emotional and physical stress of caring for a person with Alzheimer's, the center was a godsend. What a relief for me that it was so close to my home—only a few miles away.

From the moment I walked through the door for the first time, I had a good, warm feeling about the Granat Center. The facility, which occupied part of the lower level of the hospital, had a large common area for patients to color or do arts and crafts. There, too, was a large piano used for sing-alongs one afternoon a week. It also had a comfortable kitchen with a homey feel to it. Rather than industrial, the kitchen looked like one you'd see in someone's home. The most significant feature of the center, however, was the staff. From the director, Martha Wolf, on down to the aides, I got the feeling that I was surrounded by expert healthcare professionals. Instinctively, I knew this was the best place for Carmen while I was at work. Now I just had to figure out how to manage all the morning, evening, and night hours in between.

Some things were easier to deal with than others. For example, although I'd made our home as safe as possible, like locking away knives and other sharp implements, Carmen would still find something to ferret away. She would hide anything that could write, from pens and pencils to markers and crayons. I'd find a pen wrapped in tissue paper and tucked behind a sofa pillow. Hours, or at most a day after removing it from its hiding place, I'd find another one in the same place, or somewhere else. There were little stashes everywhere.

One morning, I got out of the shower to find Carmen in the bedroom, her face covered with crayon markings where make-up should go. *My beautiful Carmen.* Her lips, cheeks, and eyebrows were smeared with garish colors.

When I entered the room, she turned to me, smiling. "How do I look?"

Despite the markings, she was still undeniably beautiful, and my heart broke knowing she was trying so hard to preserve some vestige of her life. Always immaculately turned out, Carmen struggled to retain the glamour she used to wear with ease. "Hon, you look great!" I answered. "But you know what? Today's gonna be a scorcher, and I'm worried your make-up will run. Tomorrow will be a better day to put some on."

"Okay," she agreed. "If you think so." With that, she went into the bathroom to wash her face.

While incidents like these were wrenching, they were easily dealt with. It was the erratic, violent behavior that finally brought me to the Granat Center. So, I got her signed up, and then launched into the first day of our new schedule.

I felt pretty good about things at first. Day One at the Granat Center had gone off without a hitch, and I had it in my head that we could manage this. However much it wasn't what either one of us had planned, I thought Carmen and I could live a life together this way. When I arrived to pick her up that day, she'd given me a great big smile and an enormous hug, which I was happy to reciprocate.

When we got home, I didn't much feel like cooking, so we ordered in. As we waited for the food to arrive, we watched television for a while. Carmen got up to go into the kitchen for a drink, and I kept one eye on her and the other on the television. Then I realized something was wrong. I noticed she was standing at the kitchen counter, crying.

Immediately, I got up and went to the kitchen, enveloping Carmen in a soft embrace. "What's the matter hon," I whispered into her ear.

"I'm scared," she said for the first time. "I feel like you're slipping away from me and I can't stop it." She turned to face me, her eyes scanning my face. "I need you so much to get through this."

Reaching out to hold her face, I said, "I just think you're a little tired. Don't worry, I'll keep my ugly Irish mug in front of you all the time. No one could forget a face like this."

"Listen," she said, ignoring my attempt at levity. "When I get real bad and you have to put me in a nursing home—"

"Stop," I interrupted her. "I don't want to talk about that."

"No! Listen, please," she persisted, reaching up to place her hands over mine. "I'm going to keep three words for you embedded in my brain, three words I'm *not* going to let this disease have."

"What words would they be, hon?" I asked, though I already knew what they were.

"I Love You," she said firmly, her eyes locked on mine. "Whenever you hear those words, that's my signal that I know you're there."

"Okay," I said, my voice faltering. "I will remember those three words. Always."

Just then, the doorbell rang. *The food*, I thought with relief. If it hadn't been for that, I would have started balling my eyes out.

After that night, we began our new routine. Our day started at 5:00 a.m., when Carmen awoke. Though not my best hour of the day, I had no choice but to get up and on with things. Getting on with things meant, first off, conflict. I had to get Carmen into the shower and washed, which I am sure violated her sense of self-sufficiency and privacy. Though she had rapidly lost many faculties and basic skills, underneath there were still traces of familiar habits and thoughts. So, she would argue with me, and, despite my best efforts, this often led to her becoming physically violent.

After the shower, I put toothpaste on her toothbrush and oversaw that phase of the morning routine, followed by Listerine wash. Then I picked out some clothes for her to wear that day, combed her hair, and applied light make-up. I had learned to apply make-up when my grandmother was stricken with Multiple Sclerosis. She told me, "You have to do my make-up before your grandfather gets home. Even though I'm a cripple, I still have to look good for my husband." Unable to move, she delighted in having her face 'put on,' and I followed her instructions, carefully applying a light powder, eye shadow, mascara, and lipstick. It was many years later that I did the same for Carmen, so my make-up skills were rusty, but Carmen's complexion was so beautiful she didn't need much of it, and my lack of skill could never make anything less than lovely. She always called herself Patty Pale Face if she didn't powder her nose once in a while in the course of the day, so I'd always say, "All right, let's get your make-up on now. I don't want you going to the Granat Center looking like Patty Pale Face." She'd nod her approval and say "Thank you," though it was clear from her words and expression that the title was no longer familiar to her.

Once Carmen was ready, I would shower, shave, and dress as quickly as possible so as not to lose sight of her for long. Then it was time for breakfast, which typically consisted of a glass of juice, cereal, a piece of pound cake, or maybe a couple of slices of white toast, and finished off with a cup of tea. Finally, we'd head over to the center, where I'd turn her over to the staff.

Once I got Carmen safely to Granat, it was time to drive the usual thirty miles to work. Typically, I'd be at my desk no later than 9:30. I had to leave work by 4:30 in order to be back at Granat by 5:30 before they closed. Then I'd start the evening routine until it was time for Carmen to go to sleep.

As the months went by, I began to falter. Carmen began to get progressively more agitated and violent in the mornings, so that by the time we got to the Granat Center, I felt like I'd already worked an eight-hour day. In the shower alone, she'd take quite a few swings at me, and even connected a few times. *If nighttime brings 'sundowning' behavior, then this must be sunupping*, I thought, trying to duck.

The morning behavior was especially hard to handle when I'd been up all night keeping an eye on Carmen. She often became restless, and moved about the house, maybe looking for a knife or some other such object to hide. One day was especially trying. After having been up all night, I had a rough morning with Carmen. Then work was particularly hectic, so by the time I arrived at the center at 5:30 to pick Carmen up, I was barely keeping my eyes open.

I got Carmen into the car and left the parking lot to reach the main exit. The stoplight there was red, so I put my head back on the headrest for a moment while waiting for the light to change. The next thing I knew, horns were blaring behind me. I jerked awake, eyes wide open.

"Hey buddy!" a bus driver called out his window from the opposite direction. "Ya oughtta sleep at home, not here."

"Sorry," I called back, and with a half-hearted wave to the cars behind me, I accelerated through the intersection.

As I turned left out of the complex, I glanced over at Carmen, who seemed completely oblivious to what had just happened. "Hey hon," I snapped. "You could've said something." I knew I shouldn't have said anything, let alone snapped at her like that, but it just came out. I just had to blame somebody.

She just looked at me blandly and smiled. I smiled back, kicking myself mentally for yelling at a disease and expecting a person to answer.

When we pulled up to our driveway, Carmen asked, "Where are we going?"

"Into the house," I replied absent-mindedly. My tone of voice might as well have said, 'Isn't it obvious?' I should have been paying attention to what she'd said.

"That's not *my* house!" She yelled. "I'm not going in there!"

"Carmen, please," I said. "It's been a long day and I'm tired. C'mon, let's go."

"No!" she persisted, and folded her arms decisively.

Slow it down, Pat, I told myself. I knew better than to think I could make the disease see clearly that this was our house, that I was tired and not interested in dealing with it at the moment. *Think of a better way.* "Hon," I said with a smile. "I know that's not our house, but I promised."

"Promised?"

I nodded. "Yeah, I promised the people that live here that I would walk their dog while they're out of town. I can't let a dog suffer, can I?"

With that, Carmen was out of the door and heading up the steps to take the poor animal—her own Rainey—for a walk.

Wow, that really worked! Despite feeling bad about deceiving her, I was impressed. *Next time, though,* I scolded myself. *No matter how tired I am, I have to keep things smooth.* Later on I learned that Carmen was experiencing what doctors call visual agnosia, a condition in which patients are unable to recognize familiar objects.

I have to say, though, that however tired I was at the end of the workday, it was all worth it to see Carmen's face light up when I walked through the Granat Center doors. Soon, though, even that would fade away.

I thought about what Carmen had said, about her fear of losing hold of me. *What must that be like*, I wondered as I sat night after night in my chair with my friend, the darkness. *Could there be anything more horrible than to know that every-thing you love, everything you know, even your self, is slipping away?* In those moments, I think I admired Carmen more than I ever had. *She has to be the bravest, most courageous person I have ever known.*

My thoughts drifted to my grandfather, Pop, and what his situation had been with Julia. She was only in her early forties when stricken with Multiple Sclerosis, and by the time she reached age fifty, she was completely paralyzed from the neck down. Since he could not afford a nursing home, her care fell to him.

He outfitted their apartment with a hospital bed that had rubber mattresses, a bedpan, and other tools to facilitate caring for her. Every morning, Pop would pick her up and put her in a chair so he could clean everything and make up the bed with fresh sheets. Then he'd clean her, feed her breakfast, and head off to his construction job for a long day of physical labor. After returning home, he began the process all over again. He did this for ten years. All the while, all those years until she died, dear Julia knew exactly what was happening. Every day, twenty-four hours a day, she could not move, she could do nothing for herself, not even read a book. *Which is worse,* I wondered. *Losing your body or your mind?* Then there was Pop. *A giant of a man,* I thought. I'd watched him care lovingly and uncomplainingly for his wife all that time. He was my role model—they both were.

Still, I knew that I was getting worn down as a caregiver, and realized that I would be no help to Carmen in my exhausted state. Indeed, I might even be dangerous to her and others in my condition. It was true that I had won many battles for Carmen and me, but I had to admit that I was losing the war. There was no stasis to this disease; things just kept getting worse, and they'd continue to do so until—I couldn't bring myself to think of what "until" meant. Before I could figure out what to do, however, others made the decision for me.

"Do you have a minute?" Martha Wolf asked me one morning in the fall of 2003. I'd just dropped Carmen off at the center, and apparently, she was awaiting our arrival.

"Sure," I answered.

We walked back to her office and sat down. "We're seeing an increased amount of agitation with Carmen every day."

I nodded my head in agreement.

"She's pushing some of the older patients around and, as you know, since she's quite younger than they are, she's also considerably stronger."

"I understand. What do I do now?" I asked, suddenly overwhelmed by the prospect of figuring out how to do the impossible, how I could keep Carmen home during the day, or find another daycare facility. I knew the former prospect would be virtually impossible, and the latter prospect didn't even exist.

Martha smiled comfortingly, seeming to sense my despair. "You've got an appointment with Dr. Wolf-Klein on Thursday, right?"

"Yes."

"Well, let her review Carmen's current condition with you. She'll want to talk to you about Carmen's meds, and that's not my area of expertise. Maybe we can make some progress on that side of things."

"Okay," I said, relieved that I had a couple of days before embarking on the next phase of the disease's destruction.

That Thursday afternoon, Carmen and I went to the Parker Institute for a 4:00 appointment. As usual, Dr. Wolf-Klein greeted us in the examination room with an enthusiastic smile and a hug for Carmen. "My nurse is going to give Carmen a short memory test, and after that, she'll be taken down the hall for some blood tests. Then you and I will be able to talk privately for a few minutes."

"Okay," I said. "Sounds good to me."

Moments later, the nurse arrived, and started the memory test. "Okay, Carmen," she smiled. "Let's see what you can do. What day is it?"

"Saturday," Carmen said.

"What month is it?"

"January."

"Okay. Who is the President of the United States?"

"I have no idea."

"Carmen, what is your address?"

Carmen shrugged. "I really can't remember it."

"That's okay. You did great." She got up and turned to me. "Dr. Wolf-Klein will be in shortly."

I nodded. *0 for 4.* Reaching over to pat Carmen's hand, I said, "You did really good, hon."

"Did I?" she asked.

"Yup. You nailed 'em all."

Dr. Wolf-Klein appeared with an aide to take Carmen down the hall for her blood test. "Carmen," she smiled. "This gentleman is going to draw a blood sample from you. You just need to go down the hall for a minute."

After they left, Dr. Wolf-Klein closed the door and sat down across from me. "Mr. Moffett, we're going to give you a little respite for a few weeks."

"What? I don't understand." *Maybe I'm more tired than I thought.*

"Well, the last time we spoke, you mentioned that Carmen's agitation level had increased to the point of violence. And I understand from the Granat Center that Carmen's violent there, too."

"She has her moments," I responded a bit defensively. "But it's nothing I can't handle. Just tell me what we can do, and I'll do it."

"Well, I think it's time we test medications that will level off the agitation. But, it can't be done at home. These meds are quite strong. Not only that, in order to find the right combination and dosage, we have to monitor Carmen 24/7. In case there's any adverse reaction, we'll know immediately. Sometimes, two medications will be used the same day.

"Okay, where will this be done? Here?"

"No. The L.I.J. has facilities for this on the grounds. It's called the Cottage Center, which is at Hillside Hospital—just behind the Schneider Children's Hospital. There are single-level buildings that house fifteen patients each, all exclusively for the purpose of balancing their meds."

I nodded, taking it all in. "How long does it take?"

Dr. Wolf-Klein smiled. "That's where your respite comes in. It takes about three weeks to go through all the necessary steps to find just the right mixture of medications. The end result, we hope, is that we give you back a much calmer wife. And," she continued, "you need a break. You've been under a lot of pressure. Remember what I told you the first day we met? If the caregiver doesn't take care of himself, Alzheimer's can claim two victims, patient and caregiver."

"I remember," I said. "But I'm fine, really." I was lying through my teeth. I felt half dead.

"Mr. Moffett, as we have been treating Carmen, we've also been keeping an eye on you. You've lost a lot of weight, your eyes are red and puffy—clearly, you're not getting enough rest. Use the time that Carmen's at the Cottage Center to get some sleep or get away for a few days. You need it. Don't worry, Carmen will be in good hands."

I considered the benefit of medication to both Carmen and myself, and agreed. "I don't think I'll take a trip, but a few nights of solid sleep would be welcomed."

"Good," she said.

"When do we start?"

"Probably within the next ten days. I'll call you as soon as we have an opening."

"All right," I said. "I'll wait for your call."

As Carmen and I drove home that day, I started thinking about what the next few weeks would bring to our lives. I hoped everything would work out. Carmen would feel better and be safer, and we could pick up where we left off. I trusted Dr. Wolf-Klein's guidance, and was confident she had us going in the right direction. But I had also learned early on that, with Alzheimer's, life is subject to change without notice.

28

Several days after our meeting, and true to her word, Dr. Wolf-Klein called. "Hi, Mr. Moffett," she said. "I was able to make an appointment for Carmen's testing at Hillside Hospital where the Cottage Center is located."

"Good," I said. "When do we go?"

"September 17th. You should check Carmen in at 9:30 that morning."

I glanced at my calendar. "Okay, that's five days out. Good. The sooner we can get Carmen in for testing, the sooner I can have her home."

"That's the plan," Dr. Wolf-Klein said. "That's what we hope."

She gave me the number at Hillside for me to confirm the appointment, and then I got on with the business of the day. Suddenly, I felt a renewed sense of hope—not that Carmen would be cured. I was resigned to the fact of her illness, but that with medication, she would be less dangerous to herself and others. We could still share something of our lives together.

I made the day before she was to check in at the center special. After all, she would be away from home for a few weeks, and I knew the experience would be difficult for her. So, in the afternoon, I took us over to Steppingstone Park, located next to the United States Merchant Marine Academy on the Long Island Sound, and we sat on one of the benches facing the water. The breeze coming off it was brisk and refreshing—and a little chilly. I was glad I had bundled Carmen in her ski jacket. Sitting side-by-side holding hands, we gazed out over the water. Later, we ate an early dinner at La Baraka, one of our favorite French restaurants. We ordered our usual, beef Bourguignon, which reminded me of an excellent recipe Carmen had for the same dish. She used to make it every year on my birthday. *One foot in the past, one in the present. Both with Carmen. Here we are, yet we're not both here.* I tried to push the fragmented thoughts out of my mind and look forward to how things would be when Carmen came home. Though I felt guilty for relishing the thought of sleep while the doctors sorted out medications for her, I knew it wasn't going to be long. In Carmen's new world, moments were almost all she had now. *She'll be okay without me for a little while.*

Carmen was tired when we got home from dinner at 7:00 that evening. It had been a long day, but I asked her anyway if she wanted to listen to some music. "How about a dance, like we used to?" I asked.

Her eyes were sleepy, but she said, "Sure."

After putting on a slow song, I gathered her in my arms. She could only rock a little back and forth now—or maybe it was just me moving her—while her feet remained motionless on the floor. Jim Croce's "Time In A Bottle" came on next, and

I held her head close to my chest. "If I could save time in a bottle/The first thing that I'd like to do/Is to save every day/Till eternity passes away/Just to spend them with you." There was no movement from her now at all. My throat tightened and I was overcome with the terrible thought that this was our very last dance. For the rest of our lives, we would never be like we were.

"If I could make days last forever/If words could make wishes come true/I'd save every day like a treasure and then/Again, I would spend them with you." "C'mon, Carmen," I whispered into her ear, thinking she had fallen asleep in my arms. "Let's go upstairs and get you into bed."

She stirred and, without lifting her head whispered back, "No, not yet. Let's hear the rest of the song."

"Okay," I said, wiping my eyes.

She pressed her face deeper against me and we stood in the middle of the living room, listening to our life together fade away. "But there never seems to be enough time/To do the things you want to do/Once you find them/I've looked around enough to know/That you're the one I want to go/Through time with."

When the song finished, I helped Carmen upstairs and into bed. As I turned out the lights I knew tomorrow was going to be a difficult day. *It's not for long,* I consoled myself. *Not for long, and it'll be good for Carmen.*

The next morning, Carmen, P.J. and I left the house at 8:30. I was glad to have my son along for support—that's what I needed most, and he was there whenever he could be to give it. From the outside of Hillside Hospital, things looked promising. It looked to be a fairly modern facility—I didn't want

Carmen cooped up in a dingy old hospital—so I was hopeful that the inside would be just as nice. Instead of entering the hospital itself, however, we checked in at the administrative offices. But again, they looked comfortable and bright enough, so I didn't ask to see the cottage where Carmen would be staying.

It took us about forty-five minutes to get through all the paperwork with Nancy Blovian, Hillside Hospital's Senior Administrator. After she checked Carmen in, I handed over a small suitcase of clothes I'd packed for Carmen. "Okay, Mr. Moffett," she said. "We'll take her from here and get her settled in."

"Oh," I said, thinking I'd walk Carmen to her room.

For her part, Carmen suddenly realized what was happening. Her eyes widened and she looked to me for help. "Hon," I said, putting my arm around her. "This lady is going to take you for an exam, okay? And I'll see you later."

"No!" she exclaimed, her eyes pleading with me. "Don't leave me!"

"It's okay, hon. It's okay. It'll be fine. Don't worry, I'll be back in a little while."

The woman held the bag with Carmen's clothing in one hand, and reached out to her with the other. She smiled warmly, and said, "Mrs. Moffett, we're just going for some tests. It's okay."

Carmen looked back at me, and then all the nervousness just seemed to drain out of her, like she didn't have the energy for it. "Okay," she said, her voice sounding feeble. "I'll wait for you."

I watched the administrator lead Carmen away, Carmen's steps slow and careful. Once, she glanced back at me, but kept walking. I left the building as fast as I could. Seeing her leave like that made me feel like I had abandoned her. *Only three weeks,* I said over and over to myself. *Only three weeks.*

"You all right, Dad?" P.J. asked when I met up with him in the lobby.

I nodded, but didn't say anything. He went on to work, but I decided to go home. Leaving Carmen felt like a body blow. I just couldn't face going to work, where I knew I'd be good for nothing.

Rainey met me at the door when I arrived. "Hey, girl," I said wearily. She sniffed around me, then stood at the doorway looking down the street one way and then the other. I knew she was looking for her best friend, Carmen. Despite the ravages of the disease, Carmen had always been gentle with Rainey, who was her constant companion. "C'mon back inside," I said. Looking dejected, Rainey walked back to her dog bed in the living room and just stood in the middle of it. "Don't worry," I said, patting her head. "Mommy will be back soon." I had to tell myself almost the same thing later on that evening as I ate a solitary dinner. *Carmen will be back soon.*

That night, I returned to Hillside to visit Carmen. After I received my pass, I entered through the security gate that led to the hospital entrance rather than the administration building. As soon as I parked, I began to feel uneasy. Tucked behind the main administration offices and the surrounding hospital, Strauss Cottage, where Carmen was staying, was austere and industrial looking. Inside wasn't an improvement. I got to the front door and rang the bell. There was heavy glass on the front door that led to a small, dimly lit anteroom with a desk and a security guard, and another similar-looking door beyond that. A buzzer signaled the first door was now unlocked, and I entered the anteroom, where I signed the guest book. As the first door fell shut behind me with a heavy thud, I showed the guard my badge. *It's like I'm going into a prison,* I thought, feeling uncomfortable. I didn't want to think about how Carmen must be feeling inside, all alone.

The guard buzzed me through to the main room, and I immediately began looking for Carmen. I found her sitting alone in the hall, whose gray tile floors, off-white walls, and fluorescent lighting gave the feeling of being in a permanent dusk. Everything was clean, just not the least bit cheery.

As soon as she saw me, she leapt to her feet. "Hi!" she said enthusiastically. "Can I go home now?"

She broke my heart, looking at once so small and fragile, but in her excitement also almost entirely herself. "Not just yet," I answered, giving her a hug. "But it'll be soon. Let's go sit down." I guided her over to a small cafeteria area where there were four by ten foot tables. Carmen and I sat across from each other, and once again, I felt like I was on a prison visit. One of the staff brought over two Dixie cups each with small scoops of ice cream, but neither one of us was very interested. I took the ice creams and thanked the nurse. *Well, at least the staff is pleasant.*

After her initial exuberance, Carmen barely spoke. Instead, she just seemed to stare blankly at the wall-mounted television.

"Hey, hon," I said, trying to peak her interest. "Look. It's *Jeopardy.* Remember when we used to play it at home?"

"I never did that," she said, her voice dull. "You must be thinking of somebody else." Her eyes never left the screen.

I stayed with her for about an hour and then headed home, feeling a mixture of desolation and optimism. Leaving Carmen in that lifeless place was made only bearable by the fact that it was only temporary. I knew that we could weather the storm if the whole family pulled together.

29

The kids and I made a plan to visit Carmen on a rotating basis so there would be someone with her much of the time. Lesly came during the daytime on as many days as she could, Lisa brought a small picnic with Spanish food on Saturdays, and Craig, P.J., and I alternated evenings.

The first week, all I did outside of work and seeing Carmen was sleep. Then I started working out at the gym and eating better, adding more fruits and vegetables to each meal. *By the time Carmen comes home*, I thought, *we'll both be better.*

"You can't just leave her *alone* like that."

"What?" It was Lisa on the other end of the line. She called me after her first Saturday visit with Carmen.

"When we're not there. She's all alone."

"Lisa, I don't get it. She's in a hospital for *tests*. I can't be there all the time."

"Well, you could at least have someone be with her when we're not there."

"You mean like hire a sitter?"

"Right."

"You can do that?"

"Of course," she said as if it was obvious.

"Okay, I'll call the hospital." I had no idea that there were people who you could hire to spend the day with someone inside the hospital. It would be nice for Carmen to have company throughout the day.

I called the administration offices at Strauss, and they confirmed what Lisa told me. After giving me the name of an agency, I arranged for Carmen to have a sitter. Her name was Maria Warnke, a fine young lady with whom Carmen immediately bonded. Maria became like a daughter to Carmen, and I was relieved she had someone by her side when I couldn't be there.

As the third week of Carmen's stay at Strauss approached, I began to make plans for her homecoming. Though during visits I couldn't tell how the medication testing was going, I assumed the doctors were making progress. So I made sure the fridge was stocked with her favorite foods and that the house was exactly as it was when she went into the hospital.

After the third week was finished, I called the hospital. "Well, Mr. Moffett," one of the doctors there told me. "The tests are inconclusive. We need more time."

I knew that they were testing out a variety of doses and combinations of medications, and that the process was not a speedy one. So, I went about business as usual, thinking a week or two more ought to be enough. But the fifth week brought no new results. *Okay,* I thought. *Just a little more time.*

Sometime during the sixth week, a call came in to my office that changed everything forever.

"Mr. Moffett, hello. This is Nancy Blovian from Hillside

Hospital." Her voice sounded formal, as if compensating for something I couldn't pinpoint.

"Hi," I said brightly. I figured this was the call to tell me Carmen was ready to go home.

"I've got two of our psychiatrists on the call with us." They introduced themselves and said their hellos.

"Okay," I said. "Hello." I thought they were all on to instruct me on how to administer Carmen's medications. "So, what's the plan?"

"Well," one of the doctors said. "Things have not gone as well as we would have liked." He paused, perhaps waiting for a response from me. When I said nothing, he continued. "The psychopotenic drugs that seem to work for Carmen are very, very powerful."

That's good, right? Powerful drugs will help Carmen. How can he say that things weren't going as well as they wanted?

"What this means is that Carmen should not go home. We strongly recommend she live in a skilled nursing facility."

"What! How can this be?" My head started spinning. "But I was *told* you'd find the right drugs and she'd come home! You found the drugs."

"Yes, I know," the doctor agreed. His voice was sympathetic and patient. "I'm sorry to be telling you this. But the strength of the drugs is the result of all the other combinations having failed. We can't guarantee that this combination of drugs she's now on will continue to be effective. If she's taken home, she could be a danger to herself, you, or anyone she comes in contact with."

I took it all in, still dumbfounded at what I was hearing. "If the drugs stop working, we could try something else," I protested. "And anyway, it won't be worse than it is now."

"Mr. Moffett, I know this is hard to hear. It's not what you wanted or expected, and it's not what we want, either. But I promise you, it's dangerous for Carmen to live anywhere but a place that is equipped to deal with dementia illnesses like Alzheimer's. And it's not just the violence that's at issue here. These drugs are so powerful that Carmen could suffer from a seizure. If she starts convulsing in the middle of the night, and you call 9-1-1, the EMT's aren't going to know how to treat her. I'm talking about a life-threatening situation here, Mr. Moffett. Carmen could die. What I am advising you to do is not what any of us want, least of all you and Carmen, but we believe a care facility is the only way."

In that moment, my life as I knew it had ended. A trap door opened and Carmen fell through. With one phone call, it was over. I almost dropped the receiver. "Dr. Wolf-Klein said she'd be calmer," I whispered. "This isn't happening. It can't be happening."

Then Ms. Blovian said something about a list of facilities in the area that had dementia units, but I wasn't listening. I think I choked out "Thank you," before hanging up the phone, but maybe I didn't. It was all a blur.

I sat at my desk for some time, trying to understand what was happening. *Carmen is never coming home.* It was impossible. Every time I thought the words, my brain shouted *No! Impossible!* Eventually, I heard my phone ringing, and then my assistant knocking at my door. I got up and walked out the door, leaving behind my briefcase and coat. "I have to go," I said to my assistant as I lumbered by. "I'm sorry, I have to go."

"Mr. Moffett, are you all right?" she called after me. I just kept walking.

30

Carmen and I started our lives together at the Great Neck Terrace apartments over thirty years ago. Those were lean years but good ones. After all, we were together.

After I left work, I found myself at a stoplight near the apartments. They weren't on my way home, but somehow, there I was. It was the radio that reminded me. I don't recall turning it on, but it was, and the Stylistics song playing sent me back to the 1970s. *If I just went right instead of left*, I thought, *maybe I could go back to the way things were.* I envisioned walking in the door to see a smiling Carmen and three small girls rush up to greet me. *That* was life. What was happening now?

I made it home, but did not go inside right away. Instead, I sat in the car staring at the house. The living room window where I stood waiting for Carmen to come home from the store reminded me of how fast things had changed. That day was my first clue that something was wrong, but I couldn't have known it then. No one would have thought that whip smart, funny, beautiful, caring, and *young* Carmen could of all things have Alzheimer's.

There was the front door, and just beyond that the mud room. Beyond that was Carmen's kitchen, and the dining room where we celebrated so many birthdays and holidays with the wonderful Puerto Rican dishes she prepared. Just steps away was the living room where Carmen and I played along with "Jeopardy"—with Carmen always getting the question right. The living room was also our Friday night dance floor. Then, upstairs was the bedroom where we slept soundly side-by-side. *How can I go in there? I can't. I can't.* I sobbed uncontrollably. *She's never coming home. There is no more home.*

Eventually, I went inside. I knew I had to call the kids to tell them the devastating news. Five times, five hearts breaking, and mine with each one of them.

P.J. and I had been working together for some time, and so at that point was closest to day-to-day events. I decided to call him first, hoping the news would be less of a shock to him and so easiest to tell. It wasn't less shocking or easy to talk about, but P.J. understood. Like the others who I called after, he couldn't believe it. We'd all been living our lives thinking Carmen was coming home.

"What are you *talking* about?" Lisa said angrily. "You're just going to throw her away like that? I can't believe it. You're just throwing her away."

I felt like I'd just been punched in the gut. "Throwing her away? Lisa, what are *you* talking about?"

"She's not convenient anymore, so you're just going to get rid of her," Lisa snapped. I could hear her crying.

"Lisa, honey, no. You know that's not true."

"I don't *understand!*"

"Me either. None of it makes sense. But the doctors are telling me that it's too dangerous for her to live at home."

"No," she said. "I don't believe it. I don't believe it. I can't believe you'd do this to her."

"Lisa, please," I protested, my broken heart breaking into smaller and smaller pieces. "It's not like that. I'll take you to the doctors, okay? You should speak with them. They can explain it to you better than I can. Okay?"

She agreed, and I arranged to have us meet with the doctors at the Strauss cottage. P.J. and Lesly came, too. The four of us emerged from the meeting exhausted and dazed. The hopelessness of the situation was now clear to us all, even if we would not accept it for some time.

31

With a short list of nursing homes with dementia units, I started researching. We were fortunate that there were several in the area, which meant that, provided there was space at each home, I would have some choices. The people at the Strauss cottages told me that, although they would not be able to keep Carmen for a long time—after all, it was a testing facility, not a care facility—they would give the me time I needed to make arrangements for her. I knew that meant there was no time to waste. Even though Strauss' social worker gave me a list of appropriate nursing homes, the dementia unit requirement whittled down my choices considerably. For safety reasons, Alzheimer's patients had to be sequestered from the rest of the population.

I did not see Carmen right away, not only because I had to find a place for her, but I could not bear it. Though she was fading and would not know what was happening—this would be the only small consolation—I could not face her. Not yet.

Our parish priest, Monsignor Brendan Riordan, knew one of the places on my list, Our Lady of Consolation. Located on the boardwalk in West Islip, it was close to my work. I made an appointment with Sister Eileen, Consolation's director. Although there were no spaces available at the lovely facility— it looked more like a hotel than a medically outfitted nursing home—Sister Eileen offered me good advice and opened my eyes to the reality of early onset Alzheimer's. One man who would soon be coming to the home was only thirty-eight years old. Thirty-eight—and with two children. I was reminded of that saying: I complained I had no shoes until I met a man with no feet. Though Carmen's situation was no less devastating, I silently thanked God that I hadn't lost her at thirty-eight, and prayed for the man and his family—especially his two young children.

I knew a space would not open at Our Lady of Consolation, and anyway, it would be rather a far drive for the kids to visit, but I put her name on the list just in case. Then I turned my attention to the two facilities in Great Neck. Of the two of them, Wedgewood gave me a nicer feeling. It was a three-storey building laid out in such a way that there was a nice courtyard with picnic tables and plenty of room to move around and get fresh air. Fortunately, they had space, so I arranged for Carmen to be transferred there within the week. I would not be able to do it safely myself, so I arranged for an ambulance to make the fifteen minute trip, and Lesly would go with her. Now I had to go see Carmen.

It was raining that night, which contributed to the somber mood. It was the first time I was at Strauss Cottage since learning that Carmen was not coming home. Though the place never had a happy feel before, at least I felt some optimism whenever I was there—optimism that my wife would feel better and come back with me. But now I had no such hope, and the atmosphere was punishing in its desolation. We sat at the tables I had likened to a prison's visiting area, and I told Carmen that she was going to have a nice new room and a pretty courtyard. I knew I'd get no reaction, but I had to tell her. Reaching out to squeeze her hand, I told her I loved her and would always be with her. She looked at me and smiled vaguely.

I could bear no more, and got up to leave. Carmen followed me to the double glass doors, where a nurse met me. I walked into the anteroom to sign out, thinking the nurse had steered Carmen back down the hall, but something made me turn around. There was Carmen, her hands reaching for me, a pained expression on her face. Overcome with grief, I ran out the door and into my car. For thirty minutes, I sat there sobbing. I couldn't move. Everything was lost.

32

There was so much I wanted to say to her, so many things left undone and unsaid. Over the next several weeks, I seemed to stop living. I wasn't sleeping or eating, and was good for very little at work. Visits with Carmen were brutal, a constant reminder that this was her home now, but nothing could keep me from being with her.

Everything reminded me of her. I stopped watching the television, because the moment *Jeopardy!* came on, I would be overcome. Those moments hit me like a wallop on my chest. I couldn't listen to the radio, because every song reminded me of my music and dance loving Carmen. P.J. and I were still working together, and he saw my deterioration. Every night he called me to check in, and if I didn't answer the phone, there would be a knock on my door within the half hour.

One day, I came home from work early, put on a pair of shorts and a T-shirt, and drove over to my doctor's office. "Somebody help me," I said. I knew something was going to happen if I did not get help that very moment. Within an hour, I was in a psychiatrist's office. I lived, I had to live, because I could not leave Carmen alone in the world. Whatever memories the disease had stolen from her, she never has forgotten me. She doesn't know what role I play in her life, but she knows I am important to her. I will not let the disease take that from her, too.

Epilogue

As I write these words, Carmen has been in the nursing home for over three years. I visit often—typically three times a week—and always try to bring her favorite fruit, honeydew melon. On nice days, I take her out on the veranda, where we sit together at a picnic table holding hands and enjoying the fresh air together. Sometimes I find myself enjoying the moment with her so much that everything else drops away and it's just Carmen and me like we've always been. But that moment ends as soon as it's begun. I know where my beloved wife is, and I know what of her is forever lost to me—and to herself. Although she cannot understand what I am saying to her, I tell her how the kids are doing, how big her precious grandchildren are getting, how my day at the office was.

Sometimes as we sit outside holding hands, I notice the North Shore University hospital, which sits on Community Drive diagonally across from the nursing home. Somewhere inside the ten-storey glass walled building our sons, P.J. and Craig were born. I remember how happy Carmen and I were that despite the initial scare with P.J. we had healthy children. Never once had I looked out from the maternity ward windows and gave a thought about the building down below, across the street, the building where Carmen lives now. *Not in a million years would I have thought. If it was heaven up there, then I must be sitting in hell.*

I know Carmen and I aren't the only ones. I know there are tens of millions of people around the world afflicted with the disease and its effects on everyone who love them. In Carmen's family alone, Alzheimer's has destroyed the lives of three out of the four siblings. Astonishingly enough, not only do Carmen and her sister Millie have Alzheimer's, so does their brother, J.R. As I sit with Carmen at the nursing home, I wonder about them and the millions and millions of people trying to cope with this dreadful disease.

When it's just about time to end my visit, I walk Carmen to the elevator and back to her room. We walk slowly, not just because she has to. I don't want to hurry.

I always ask one of the aides to be available when we arrive back at Carmen's room to distract her so I can slip out the door so she can forget me until our next visit. Truth be told, I always have difficulty leaving her. It has never ceased being overwhelmingly emotional for me. So, as the aide gently holds her arm to steer her into her room, I kiss her lightly on the forehead and turn to leave.

Despite everything Carmen has been through, despite the way this terrible disease has robbed her of herself, her life, and our lives together, this beautiful and amazing woman has not forgotten the three words she saved just for me. Sometimes, as I turn to leave, I hear her say, "I love you."

I whisper back, "I love you, too."

Appendix I: The Future of Alzheimer's
By
Dr. Gisele Wolf-Klein, M.D.
Chief, Division of Geriatric Medicine
Long Island Jewish Medical Center

As this book went to press, approximately 4.5 million Americans were afflicted with Alzheimer's disease. Worldwide, the percentage of people with this dreadful disease was estimated at 24.3 million people. Researchers believe that, by 2050, the number will reach 14 million in the United States, and a staggering 80 million throughout the World. Quite simply, there won't be enough beds—not enough care facilities—to cope with this volume of dementia patients.

But long before we reach 2050, the projected number of Alzheimer's patients in America is expected to explode. This projection is based in large part on the so-called "baby boomer" generation, those 76 million people born between 1946 and 1964. These "Geri-boomers" are often well-educated, financially secure, married, and with children. They have ready access to information through media and Internet networks. Nevertheless, a recent study conducted through the Long Island Jewish Medical Center/Geriatric Fellowship found that these "boomers" have "unrealistic expectations of the current health system." What this means is that even the people who might be considered most savvy about their own geriatric care are not educated enough on "the financial realities of aging." Worse yet, the number of physicians specializing in geriatric care is not increasing with the number of patients who will need their services. When situated in the context of Alzheimer's care, American "baby boomers" the study's results are frightening. In a few short years, more people than ever will be diagnosed with Alzheimer's disease, but be little prepared for what's in store.

The disabilities that result from Alzheimer's disease are many and varied. From initial memory loss and confusion to debilitating pain and the inability to care for oneself, the nature of the disability presents special burdens for Alzheimer's patients, their caregivers, and researchers working to find new therapies.

At present, though there are treatments available that target the symptoms of the disease, there is no cure. Acetylcholinesterase agents are the most common drugs administered to Alzheimer's patients. But while these medications help to decrease the symptoms of mild to moderate Alzheimer's, they don't help everyone with the disease, especially those in whom the disease has entered its more advanced stages. Another version of the acetylcholinesterase agent helps prevent deterioration in moderate to severe cases of Alzheimer's, but again, it's not universally successful. There is also evidence that anti-inflammatory drugs like ibuprofen are helpful in slowing the progression of the disease, and there are experimental drugs currently in clinical trials that may soon make their way to the marketplace.

One experimental drug that initially seemed promising directly attacked the molecule, amyloid peptide, that accumulates in the brain like a plaque, slowing down the progress of the disease. (Whether or not this plaque and tangles of abnormal filaments of the protein tau are symptoms or causes of the disease is not known.) However, it's efficacy is now doubted. In addition, a vaccine called intravenous immunoglobulin (IVIg) may be efficacious for people known to be predisposed to the disease. The drug has the potential to wipe out the disease, which, given the staggering figures listed above, could be a monumental advance in Alzheimer's research. In addition, early detection techniques, such as the PET scan, also appear to be promising. By imaging changes in healthy older people, researchers could begin to formulate physical signs of Alzheimer's earlier than the behavioral symptoms that presently signal the onset of the disease. Annual volumetric imaging is a procedure that compares yearly brain scans, revealing decreases in the size of the part of the brain called the hippocampus. Such decreases correlate with the development of Alzheimer's.

Despite the progress researchers have made, there is no cure on the horizon, and many people suffering from the disease will not be helped by the newest medications, either because the disease is too far along for such therapy, or because in some individuals, the disease seems to be resistant to it.

What is particularly tragic about Alzheimer's is the way in which the disease inexorably destroys brain tissue, and along with it, the patient's cognitive functions, such as memory, language, and self-awareness, and they suffer terrible mood disorders. Eventually, they lose physical capacities, and concomitant illness, such as pneumonia, typically end the life of someone with Alzheimer's—yet their lives were effectively finished before death finally comes to claim them.

As the numbers of Alzheimer's patients increase, and younger and younger patients are diagnosed with the disease, the burden will be unbearable unless we dramatically increase the funding for Alzheimer's therapy research and training of Alzheimer's specialists. The future is clear, and the time to act is now.

Appendix II: Selecting a Caregiver

When I knew I had to find a caregiver to help me with Carmen's daily care, I wasn't sure how to proceed. I'd been given a list of agencies by the Parker Institute, but there was no direction as to how to find someone suitable for Carmen. The choice of who will care for your loved one is fraught with worry. After all, the caregiver will be spending significant numbers of hours every week in your home with someone very dear to you, and will be privy to the details of your life. Ideally, you'd want a caregiver to be someone close to you, someone both you and the patient can trust immediately. The optimum situation would be to have a caregiver that is a close friend or relative, not only because they would be trustworthy, but also because they may know some of the history of the patient. In addition, the caregiver automatically feels a sense of deep responsibility to, and comfort with, the patient. Unfortunately, however, it's not always possible to make the sort of long-term arrangement required for Alzheimer's care.

What makes most people nervous about working with an outside caregiver is that you don't really know whom you're accepting into your home. However, if you are faced with going outside your circle of trusted family and friends, you may want to go to your local religious community as they may be able to recommend a volunteer program. You can also check with the local Alzheimer's Association chapter, who will be able to recommend a home care agency. Whether it's a volunteer or an agency remember you're inviting a stranger into the home of the patient, which can be a little unnerving. Therefore, it is important to interview the caregiver so you can reach your own comfort level with the person.

I recommend you use basic business interviewing techniques at the very least. When a salesperson visits my office, there are two things I take note of right away. The first is the handshake. It must be firm—not necessarily strong, but at least confident. Second, the individual has to look me straight in the eye. When I'm interviewing an applicant, the first impression made is important. The way a person is dressed tells me they are organized and interested in the position enough to take care of their appearance. It's not that a caregiver should be dolled up, but they should look presentable, not sloppy or disheveled.

If you're using an outside agency for caregiving services, the individuals on the agency's roster have been pre-screened. Nevertheless, since there is a high turnover rate, it is important that you watch closely who comes and goes in this long caregiving process. In addition, make sure you understand the levels of caregiving certifications and what your insurance company policy covers. Bear in mind that home care agencies charge between $15.00 and $25.00 an hour, and this is generally not covered under standard insurance policies. A CNA (certified nursing assistant) is a caregiver who is certified to work at a nursing facility, and so has the skills requisite to provide an Alzheimer's patient with preliminary emergency medical care. In fact, it's the level of certification required to work at such a facility. The next level is the HHA (home health aide). An individual with this level of certification can dispense medications, lift the patient, and provide the basic feeding and bathing caregiving duties. The lowest caregiving level is the PCA (personal care assistant), and this certification restricts caregiving duties to bathing and feeding. Depending on what your Alzheimer's patient requires, be sure to accept nothing less than the highest level of certification you can find.

Alzheimer's Disease Organizations, Resources, and Books

Organizations
Alzheimer's Association
225 North Michigan Ave., Fl. 17
Chicago, IL 60601-7633
Ph: 312-335-8700 Fax: 312-335-1110
Toll-free: 1-800-272-3900
www.alz.org

Alzheimer Society of Canada
20 Eglinton Avenue W. Suite 1200
Toronto, ON M4R 1K8
Ph: 416-488-8772 Fax: 416-488-3778
Toll-free: 1-800-616-8816
www.alzheimer.ca

Resources
The Alzheimer's Store
"The Alzheimer's Store is dedicated to providing unique products and information for those caring for someone with Alzheimer's disease. Every product in the store has been carefully selected to make living with Alzheimer's disease as easy as possible."
http://www.alzstore.com/

Well Spouse Association
63 West Main St. Suite H
Freehold, NJ 07728
Ph: 1-800-838-0879
www.wellspouse.org

National Institute on Aging
Building 31, Room 5C27
31 Center Drive, MSC 2292
Bethesda, MD 20892
Ph: 301-496-1752
www.nia.nih.gov/alzheimers

Alzheimer's Disease Education and Referral Center (ADEAR)
P.O. Box 8250
Silver Spring, MD 20907-8250
Ph: 301-495-3311 or 800-438-4380
www.alzheimers.org/adear

Alzheimer's Disease International
64 Great Suffolk Street
London, SE1 0BL
United Kingdom
Ph: 44 207 981 0880
www.alz.co.uk

American Association of Homes and Services for the Aging
2519 Connecticut Ave. N.W.
Washington, DC 20008-1520
Ph: 202-783-2242
www.aahsa.org

Centers for Medicare and Medicaid Services
7500 Security Blvd.
Baltimore, MD 21244-1850
Ph: 410-786-3000
www.cms.hhs.gov

Family Caregiver Alliance
180 Montgomery Street, Ste. 1100
San Francisco, CA 94104
Ph: 415-434-3388
www.caregiver.org

National Council on the Aging
409 Third St. S.W., Suite 200
Washington, DC 20024
Ph: 202-479-1200
www.ncoa.org

National Hospice and Palliative Care Organization
1700 Diagonal Road, Suite 625
Alexandria, VA 22314
Ph: 703-837-1500
www.nhpco.org

Long Island Alzheimer's Foundation
5 Channel Drive
Port Washington, New York 11050
Ph: 1-866-780-5423
www.liaf.org

Books
DeBaggio, Thomas. *Losing My Mind: An Intimate Look at Life With Alzheimer's.* New York: Free Press, 2002.

Hamdy, R.C., J.M. Turnbull, W. Clark and M. Lancaster. *Alzheimer's Disease: A Handbook for Caregivers.* St. Louis, Missouri: Mosby, 1994.

Hodgson, Harriet. *Alzheimer's–Finding the Words*. Minneapolis: Chronimed, 1995.

Mace, N., and P. Rabins. The *Thirty-Six Hour Day*. Baltimore: Johns Hopkins, 1981.

Temes, Roberta. *Living With an Empty Chair: A Guide Through Grief*. New York: Irvington, 1984.

Susik, H. *Hiring Home Caregivers*. San Luis Obispo, CA: Impact Publishers, 1995.

Barg, G. *The Fearless Caregiver: How to Get the Best for Your Loved One and Still Have a Life of Your Own*. Hendon, VA: Capital Books, 2001.
Kushner, H.S. *When Bad Things Happen to Good People*. New York: Avon Books, 1981.

Bridges, B.J. *Therapeutic Caregiving: A Practical Guide for Caregivers of Persons With Alzheimer's and Other Dementia-Causing Diseases*. Mill Creek, WA: BJB Publishing, 1995.

Witrogen-Mcleod, B. Caregiving: *The Spiritual Journey of Love, Loss and Renewal*. New York: John Wiley & Sons, 1999.